Play for Health Across the Lifespan

Play for Health Across the Lifespan uses case studies to explore the impact of play and creativity on health and wellbeing throughout the lifecycle. While play at the start of life influences future development, the authors show play also has a role in improving prospects for health and wellbeing in adulthood and later life.

A relational approach to health and wellbeing emphasizes the dynamic, mutually influential relationship between individual development and the changing contexts of our lives. Our personal play history is one feature of this dynamic process, and this book explores how the experience of play throughout the life course sculpts and resculpts the shape of our lives: our physical health, our mental wellbeing, and our relationship to the people and the world around us. Storytelling has been used since the beginning of time to communicate important life lessons in an engaging way. Taking inspiration from Shakespeare's 'Seven Ages of Man', the book uses a case-story approach to differentiate the stages of development and to present evidence for how play and playful experiences impact on health and wellbeing from birth to the end of life in the context of temporal and situational change. Each chapter in *Play for Health Across the Lifespan* introduces relevant evidence-based research on play and health, before presenting several narrative 'case stories', which illustrate the application of play theory and the neuroscience of play as they relate to each life stage.

With contributions from specialists in health and education, community organizations and the creative and performing arts, this book will appeal to academics, students, and practitioners who are interested in exploring the role of play in addressing contemporary challenges to our physical, mental, and social health.

Julia Whitaker has a background in social work, family therapy, and healthcare play specialism and has over 30 years' practice and teaching experience in both public and private sectors. She is currently interested in exploring how play and playfulness impact on health and wellbeing throughout the life course and has a special interest in the role of play in the attachment process.

Alison Tonkin looks after the Higher Education provision at Stanmore College, teaching and managing a range of courses linked to working with children and young people and healthcare for adults. With a research background in health promotion among preschool children and having worked as a diagnostic and therapeutic radiographer, the link between health and education is actively promoted. The importance of play and playfulness for health and wellbeing for children and adults alike is an area of particular interest.

Play for Health Across the Lifespan

Stories from the Seven Ages of Play

Julia Whitaker and Alison Tonkin

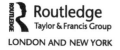

Routledge
Taylor & Francis Group

LONDON AND NEW YORK

First published 2021
by Routledge
2 Park Square, Milton Park, Abingdon, Oxon OX14 4RN

and by Routledge
605 Third Avenue, New York, NY 10158

Routledge is an imprint of the Taylor & Francis Group, an informa business

British Library Cataloguing-in-Publication Data
A catalogue record for this book is available from the British Library

Library of Congress Cataloging-in-Publication Data
A catalog record for this book has been requested

ISBN: 978-0-367-47287-0 (hbk)
ISBN: 978-0-367-47288-7 (pbk)
ISBN: 978-1-003-03469-8 (ebk)

Typeset in Bembo
by Apex CoVantage, LLC

In memory of Melanie:
a very special friend
J.W.

To Jenni and Debs:
for sharing the onerous responsibility of
Ball Duty with such love
and kindness
A.T.

Contents

Figures

Tables

Boxes

Foreword

In 2019, I gave a talk about the University of Portsmouth's Student Book Club and the strong evidence linking reading for pleasure with learning, empowerment, confidence, empathy, and health and wellbeing. After the talk, I met up with Alison Tonkin (who looks after Higher Education at Stanmore College) and we had a conversation that focused on two aspects of the talk – the therapeutic benefits of shared reading (where the reading is punctuated by personal responses) and telling stories to promote mutual understanding and quality of life. When, a year later, Alison described a book in the making that would use a case-story approach to explore health and wellbeing across the lifespan, I was pleased to be invited to write this Foreword.

Learning Developers in Higher Education use a wide range of approaches to empower students to become confident learners, including the use of storytelling as a means of sense-making. There is a strong relationship between storytelling and play which are, arguably, inseparable. Paley (1990: 4) argues that 'play is story in action, just as storytelling is play put into narrative form'. *Play for Health Across the Lifespan: Stories from the Seven Ages of Play* emphasizes the importance of play throughout the different stages of life and the interconnectedness between play and positive health. The book fittingly uses part of an extremely well-known narrative – the 'Seven Ages of Man' monologue from Shakespeare's *As You Like It* – to consider the relevance of play from our first breath to our last. The chapters are united in a conviction that storytelling and play, at any stage of life, have the potential to impact positively on the quality of life.

This book's use of a case-story approach is relevant and timely. As Tahir Shah (2008), in *In Arabian Nights: A Caravan of Moroccan Dreams*, so astutely observed, 'stories are a communal currency of humanity'. As we move from place to place, or age to age, we can experience the transformative potential of the interweaving of storytelling and play. This helps us understand our world and our place in it, in ways which would be very different if we did not have this lens to look through.

For anybody interested in the power of play and its application to health and wellbeing, *Play for Health Across the Lifespan: Stories from the Seven Ages of Play* provides a springboard for further exploration. It was Philip Pullman (2004) who talked about the 'democracy' of reading and the 'to-and-fro' between the reader and the writer. So it is with storytelling and with play, both of which invite us to be fully present, curious and, above all, involved. This book is a testament to the democracy of storytelling and play.

After all, we are, all of us, life's storytellers and players.

Rhiannon Parry Thompson is a Learning Development Tutor in the Faculty of Humanities and Social Sciences at the University of Portsmouth. In this role, she uses storytelling to support students to develop their academic voice.

References

Paley, A. (1990) *The Boy Who Would Be a Helicopter: The Uses of Storytelling in the Classroom.* Cambridge, MA: Harvard University Press.

Pullman, P. (2004) *The War on Words.* Online. HTTP: <www.theguardian.com/books/2004/nov/06/usa.politics> (accessed 26 November 2020).

Shah, T. (2008) *In Arabian Nights: A Caravan of Forgotten Dreams.* London: Bantam.

Acknowledgments

Lizzy Mikietyn, for another lively cover illustration and for interpreting our somewhat opaque instructions with such skill and patience.

Rhiannon Parry Thompson and Laura Barclay from the Learning Development Team at the School of Languages and Applied Linguistics, University of Portsmouth, whose Foreword eloquently endorses the case-story approach adopted in this book.

All the contributors to the book who have enriched this project through the generous sharing of their experience and expertise:

Alison Hawkins, *Principal, Wester Coates Nursery School, Edinburgh*

Alistair Pugh, *Teacher, Edinburgh Steiner School*

Bethany Whiteside, *Research Lecturer and Doctoral Degrees Coordinator, Royal Conservatoire of Scotland*

Carla Roberts, *Senior Workflow Administrator*

Cathy Treadaway, *Professor of Creative Practice, Cardiff Metropolitan University; founder member of CARIAD (Centre for Applied Research in Inclusive Arts and Design); Academic Lead Investigator LAUGH EMPOWERED PSCI project: www.laughproject.info*

Christina Freeman, *Radiographer (retired)*

Claire Weldon, *Student Welfare Officer*

Cristina Grohmann, *College Student*

Debbie Tonkin, *Business Manager, Cicely Saunders Institute, King's College London*

Elizabeth Henderson, *Early Years Consultant*

Elizabeth Wilkinson, *Play Therapist*

Emilie Capulet, *Senior Lecturer and Head of Classical Performance Studies, London College of Music, University of West London*

Eric Fleming, *Manager and Craft-based Educator, Seòl Trust, East Lothian, Scotland*

Erin, *Middle School Student*

Gavin Cullen, *Nurse Lecturer, Edinburgh Napier University; former Charge Nurse in a Child and Adolescent Mental Health Service*

Hilary Long, *Early Years Consultant; former Manager, Woodland Outdoor Kindergartens, Glasgow*

Ike C. Odina, *Mentor, Mentors Inspiratus . . . ! !*

Impact Arts, *community arts organization which uses the arts and creativity to enable and empower social change throughout Scotland:* www.impactarts.co.uk/

Irene Lawrence, *Retiree*

Jan Cameron, *Author of The Garden Cure (2020) Salford: Saraband*

Jenni Etchells, *Practice Education Facilitator in primary care*

Jenny Oliver, *registered Health Play Specialist, University College Hospital London*

Jo Vigar, *Deputy Care Home Manager*

Julia Findon, *Music Teacher; former Cub Scout Leader*

Kath Evans, *Director of Children's Nursing/Chair of the Children's Board, Barts Health; Nursing and Academic Fellow, School of Health Sciences, City University; Children and Young People's Clinical Lead, East London Health and Care Partnership*

Kathrine Jebsen-Moore, *Freelance Writer and Journalist*

Laura Walsh, *Head of Play Services, Great Ormond Street Hospital*

Layla Tree, *Woven Textile Designer and Workshop Leader*

Lisa Sinclair, *Dance Health Manager, Scottish Ballet*

Lorraine Close, *Director, Edinburgh Community Yoga:* https://edinburghcommunityyoga.co.uk/

Nick Hillier, *Director of Communications, Academy of Medical Sciences*

Nisi Conyngham, *Artist*

Patrick Boxall, *Forest College Co-ordinator, Newbattle Abbey College*

Sonny G. C. McLeod, *High School Student*

Starcatchers, *Scotland's National Arts and Early Years Organization:* www.starcatchers.org.uk/

Victoria Kim Webster, *Trainee Teacher*

All the photographers and their subjects, whose images tell stories of their own:

Hilary Long: Figure 3.1

Julia Findon: Figures 4.3 and 7.4

Sarah Miller: Figure 5.1 (Dominic and Iona)

Jenny Oliver: Figure 6.1

Alison Tonkin: Figures 6.2 and 9.1

Emilie Capulet: Figure 6.3

Leigh Bishop Photography: Figure 7.2 (Nisi Conyngham)

Eric Fleming: Figure 7.3

Rachel McEwen: Figure 8.1

Andy Ross Images: Figure 8.2 (Jim and Angela)

Ashley Bingham for the Liminal Space: Figures 9.2 and 9.3

Grace Etchells for the use of her drawing in Figure 4.1

Natalie Close at Spectrum Health and Training on behalf of Gooey Brains for the use of Figure 1.1

Nina Hersher on behalf of the Digital Wellness Collective for the use of Figure 5.2

Grace McInnes, Commissioning Editor at Routledge, for giving us the opportunity to take a different approach to our exploration of the links between play and health

Evie Lonsdale, Editorial Assistant, for her ready availability and for guiding us effortlessly through the publishing process

Debbie Tonkin, for once again being our diligent proofreader

Nicola Conibear and the Senior Leadership Team at Stanmore College who enabled this project to be undertaken and completed under their stewardship

Julia would like to thank

Alison, for being willing to take a different route and for trusting me to take the reins.

Freya, for a very good idea. Alex, whose hard work makes it possible for me to indulge in these scholarly pursuits.

Alison would like to thank

Julia, how lovely to watch you lead this wonderful project . . . the apprentice has become the master.

My family and Mark, whose significance and importance have been emphasized even more in these extraordinary times.

Introduction

All the world's a stage,
And all the men and women merely players;
They have their exits and their entrances;
And one man in his time plays many parts,
His acts being seven ages. At first the infant,
Mewling and puking in the nurse's arms;
And then the whining school-boy, with his satchel
And shining morning face, creeping like snail
Unwillingly to school. And then the lover,
Sighing like furnace, with a woeful ballad
Made to his mistress' eyebrow. Then a soldier,
Full of strange oaths, and bearded like the pard,
Jealous in honour, sudden and quick in quarrel,
Seeking the bubble reputation
Even in the cannon's mouth. And then the justice,
In fair round belly with good capon lin'd,
With eyes severe and beard of formal cut,
Full of wise saws and modern instances;
And so he plays his part. The sixth age shifts
Into the lean and slipper'd pantaloon,
With spectacles on nose and pouch on side;
His youthful hose, well sav'd, a world too wide
For his shrunk shank; and his big manly voice,
Turning again toward childish treble, pipes
And whistles in his sound. Last scene of all,
That ends this strange eventful history,
Is second childishness and mere oblivion;
Sans teeth, sans eyes, sans taste, sans everything.
(Shakespeare 2006 2.7: 227–228)

This book of stories starts with its own story. In the early months of 2019, well before the transition to a post-pandemic 'new normal' way of living and working, Julia's daughter came up with the suggestion that we write our next book on the subject of 'play through the ages'. This fledgling historian envisaged a chronology of play and games since ancient times, but her proposition awakened instead the notion of a personal 'play history', linked not only to an individual's developmental profile but to the social context of their playing. It is from our growing interest in this idea of our 'play history', and how it influences our health and wellbeing, that this book has emerged — with a nod to William Shakespeare.

Everyone likes a good story, and we know from our conversations, presentations, and writing about play that what people remember and want to talk about are the anecdotes and case studies that we have used to illustrate the content of our teaching and writing. We also meet an increasing number of people who have embraced the idea that play adds an extra dimension to their lives and to their work — and that they 'feel better' for it. We decided to invite some of these experts in the field to share their individual perspectives as a way of adding color to our examination of play for health, not 'through the ages' but 'through the stages' of the life course.

Much has been written about the importance of play in the lives of children: for their health and development and for their learning. In this book, we have endeavored to extend the play conversation to include its role in lifespan development, presenting the evidence for play as a universal contributory factor to health and development from birth to old age and death. This is a conversation begun five years ago in *Play in Healthcare for Adults* (Tonkin and Whitaker 2016), in which we made the case for play and playfulness as a route to positive health for those living with, or recovering from, physical or mental health challenges.

In *Play for Health Across the Lifespan: Stories from the Seven Ages of Play*, we adopt a lifespan perspective on play and health which recognizes that development is lifelong and that change is evident throughout the life stages. We acknowledge that health and development are multidirectional, with gains matched by losses across all dimensions of growth — physical, cognitive, and psychosocial — and that change in any one of these areas prompts change elsewhere (Lally and Valentine-French 2019). We celebrate the plasticity of the human brain and how it makes all things possible, given the right circumstances. We also acknowledge that our experiences change us as we move through life and that our play history contributes to that change.

A lifespan perspective is a normative approach: at each stage of human development, there are certain characteristics, experiences, and challenges which we all share. There are also historical and cultural commonalities in the way we live and how our health is impacted by our location in time and in society. However, a lifespan model must also allow for the fact that the unique experiences and circumstances of our individual lives influence us in different ways. Human health and development are complex, dynamic processes which function with the purpose of 'enlarging people's freedoms and opportunities and improving their well-being' (Social Science Research Council 2020). To live a healthy life is not an end in itself; the value of 'good health' lies in the fact that 'like money, it is a prerequisite for a decent, fulfilling life' (O'Mahony 2016).

Playing with history

Two actual historical considerations have found their way into the writing of this book.

Referencing Shakespeare's (2006) 'Seven Ages of Man' in the title and structure of this book has required a degree of artistic license in order to make our stories fit into seven life stages. At the time of Shakespeare's writing at the end of the sixteenth century, children leapfrogged straight from '*mewling infancy*' to school, missing out entirely on our transitional 'Early Years' – which we have incorporated in our first life stage (Chapter 3). Shakespeare's '*schoolboy*' then made a swift transition to the stature of '*lover*' and, while modern-day adolescents may still frequently '*sigh like a furnace*', they have more and better reasons for doing so than a broken heart. And young adults in twenty-first-century Britain have many options for making their mark on society, other than success in battle. Many of today's baby-boomers certainly display the same '*round belly*' as Shakespeare's Justice; and those of us approaching our '*sixth age*' indeed have spectacles on our noses, even if our shanks have not shrunk! However, in Shakespeare's day, few people would have reached his last stage of '*second childishness*' whereas the fastest growing age group in the UK are the over-85s (Age UK 2019), whom we celebrate in our last life stage (Chapter 9).

Shakespeare's finest writing coincided with a period of great personal and social anguish and upheaval. As the Black Plague swept through Europe during the sixteenth century, its impact reverberated in both his private and professional life. Three of Shakespeare's sisters and his young son died from the plague and his plays are littered with references which reflect 'an awareness about how precarious life can be in the face of contagion and social breakdown' (Yachnin 2020). Theatres were the first public spaces to be locked down during peaks in infection, and between 1603 and 1613 Shakespeare's Globe was closed for a total of 78 months (Ainley 2020): the playwright would certainly have been familiar with the challenges of living and working in a state of uncertainty and change.

Jump to the present day. We could not have imagined when we signed with Routledge in January 2020 that, within three months, we too would be living through a time of dread and fear which would see us all 'locked-down' in our respective homes and countries. The repercussions of the Covid-19 coronavirus pandemic of 2020 have once again brought into stark focus the human need for adaptability and highlighted the complex relationship between our health (physical and mental) and other aspects of our lives. In the shadow of daily reports of increased hospitalizations and deaths, we have seen a resurgence of play as a catalyst for change. Unable to leave the home for work or school, many people rediscovered – or discovered for the first time – the joy of play, through music-making, singing, dancing, reading, crafting, painting, walking with no exterior motive other than to find pleasure and meaning in a different way of living (Tonkin and Whitaker 2020). This book is not about play in a pandemic but its central tenet, that play is good for you, reinforces what many people have learned during the unprecedented circumstances of 2020.

Defining terms

Chapter 1 examines how definitions of play have evolved over time and addresses the ongoing debate about whether play is always necessarily 'playful'. As in our previous books (Tonkin and Whitaker 2016, 2019), play is differentiated according to three defining characteristics borrowed from Bateson (2014) and others. The tripartite definition of play used throughout this book describes an activity or disposition which is *intrinsically motivated, personally rewarding*, and which *values process over outcome*. In the following chapters, the reader will encounter descriptions of attitudes and behaviors which may challenge their own perceptions of play; we hope only to stimulate dialogue and further inquiry.

Just as our understanding of the nature of play has changed over time, so is the case for the concept of 'health'. No longer regarded as simply the absence of disease, it is now widely accepted that a healthy life incorporates aspects of the social and environmental – as well as the physical and mental state. A recognition that positive health derives from an ability to adapt and cope with changes in one's person and in one's life circumstances acknowledges the overlap between the different aspects of our lives and allows for consideration of a wider range of measures for promoting and nurturing health and for responding to health challenges as they arise (Health Knowledge 2017).

Why stories?

Chapter 2 sets out the argument in favor of storytelling as a valid tool for conveying important messages about how to live a good and healthy life. It starts with an overview of the ways in which stories have been used throughout history to communicate information, to empathize with different aspects of the human predicament, and to offer succor in times of trouble. The chapter goes on to explore the use of a narrative model for knowledge development in a professional context, for challenging preconceptions, and for prompting change.

The case-story approach, which lies at the heart of this book, offers readers the opportunity to hear from a wide range of contributors who have generously agreed to share their own perspectives on play 'for health's sake'. Each of our contributors was invited to tell their story using their own voice which has resulted in a rich tapestry of different styles, ranging from the deeply personal narrative to the more academic reflection and evaluation.

The seven ages

In the words of Shakespeare (2006), we '*play many parts*' during our time on this earthly stage, and how and what we play changes with life's seasons. Chapters 3 to 9 take the reader through our 'Seven Ages of Play' – from infancy and the early years, through childhood, adolescence, early, middle, and older adulthood to the end of life.

Our human story begins with the brain and each of these chapters begins with an overview of brain development at the different life stages, exposing the symbiotic relationship between what is happening in the brain and our health status – and how play can be a mediator in this process. This is not a new idea: over 2000 years ago, Hippocrates (cited in Swaab 2015: 3) declared that 'It should be widely known that the brain, and the brain alone, is the source of our pleasures, joys, laughter and amusement, as well as our sorrow, pain, grief and tears'. However, the evolution of our scientific knowledge and understanding means that we now recognize that the human brain is created 'remarkably unfinished' (Eagleman 2015: 6), allowing it to adapt to, and to be shaped by, our personal experience of the world. The brain is indeed the source of our play, but it is also replenished by our playing.

At each life stage, we have isolated themes of specific health concern using the case-stories to enhance discussion of relevant theory and research. In a book of this size, the themes are clearly selective and reflect our own areas of interest and expertise: we recognize that there are many others still to explore.

Chapter 3: Infancy and the early years looks at play as a mediator in the processes of early attachment and separation and at the role of play in nature for evoking the senses of awe and wonder which inspire the child's curiosity, joy, and engagement with the world.

Chapter 4: The school years addresses the relationship between play and education and considers the latest research into the impact of screen use in childhood.

Chapter 5: Adolescence reframes the teenage years as a positive life stage and proposes that play has a crucial role in the nurture of lifelong passions and a sense of purpose in life.

Chapter 6: Early adulthood examines the link between play and creativity and the role of playfulness in adult relationships.

Chapter 7: The middle years discusses the concept of work–life balance and looks at how play can nurture wellbeing in the middle years and offer a creative route to mental health.

Chapter 8: Elderhood tackles the problem of loneliness in old age and discusses the ways in which play can enhance physical, mental, and social health and wellbeing.

Chapter 9: The end of life introduces the concept of super-aging, before going on to discuss the link between play and the realization of authenticity at life's ending.

We hope this book will be of interest to a broad readership, most obviously to professionals and students in the fields of health, social care, and education but also to anyone who is interested in incorporating play and playfulness in their life and in their work. Recognizing the contribution made by play to our health and development invites further examination of the concept of a personal 'play history' and greater advocacy for play opportunities at all stages of the life course.

Hanson (2013: 39) writes that 'mammals, including us, become friendly, playful, curious, and creative when they feel safe, satisfied, and connected'. In times of uncertainty and change, play is our safe place. It offers comfort, distraction, and opportunity when other sources of satisfaction are denied us. When we feel cut off from all that is familiar, it creates a connection to others and to the world in which we live. In our fast-changing world, the human propensity for play is a constant which lies at the core of our ability to adapt to change, challenge, and adversity. Today, play is more important than ever before, 'crucial for togetherness in our communities and for bridging over contradictions in our culture' (Hännikainen et al. 2013). A better future, built on a culture of health, needs to have play at the heart of its history.

References

Age UK (2019) *Later Life in the United Kingdom*. Online. HTTP: <www.ageuk.org.uk/globalassets/age-uk/documents/reports-and-publications/later_life_uk_factsheet.pdf> (accessed 31 August 2020).

Ainley, O. (2020) *Shakespeare and Plague: How Did Disease Influence the Playwright?* Online. HTTP: <www.whatsonstage.com/ballymena-theatre/news/shakespeare-plague-disease-influence_51308.html> (accessed 5 November 2020).

Bateson, P. (2014) Playfulness and creativity. *Animal Behavior and Cognition*, 1 (2): 99–112.

Eagleman, D. (2015) *The Brain*. Edinburgh: Canongate Books.

Hännikainen, M., Singer, E. and van Oers, B. (2013) Promoting play for a better future. *European Early Childhood Education Research Journal*, 21 (2): 165–171.

Hanson, R. (2013) *Hardwiring Happiness: The New Brain Science of Contentment, Calm, and Confidence*. London: Rider.

Health Knowledge (2017) *Section 3: Concepts of Health and Wellbeing*. Online. HTTP: <www.healthknowledge.org.uk/public-health-textbook/medical-sociology-policy-economics/4a-concepts-health-illness/section2/activity3> (accessed 15 November 2020).

Lally, M. and Valentine-French, S. (2019) *Lifespan Development: A Psychological Perspective*. 2nd Ed. Online. HTTP: <http://dept.clcillinois.edu/psy/LifespanDevelopment.pdf> (accessed 18 August 2020).

O'Mahony, S. (2016) *The Way We Die Now*. London: Head of Zeus Ltd.

Shakespeare, W. (2006) *As You Like It*. London: The Arden Shakespeare, Third Series.

Social Science Research Council (2020) *About Human Development*. Online. HTTP: <https://measureofamerica.org/human-development/> (accessed 18 August 2020).

Swaab, D. (2015) *We Are Our Brains: From the Womb to Alzheimer's*. London: New York.

Tonkin, A. and Whitaker, J. (Eds.) (2016) *Play in Healthcare for Adults*. Oxon: Routledge.

Tonkin, A. and Whitaker, J. (Eds.) (2019) *Play and Playfulness for Public Health and Wellbeing*. Oxon: Routledge.

Tonkin, A. and Whitaker, J. (2020) *Play and Playfulness for Health and Wellbeing: A Panacea for Mitigating the Impact of Coronavirus (COVID 19)*. Online. HTTP: <http://dx.doi.org/10.2139/ssrn.3584412> (accessed 15 September 2020).

Yachnin, P. (2020) *After the Plague, Shakespeare Imagined a World Saved from Poison, Slander and the Evil Eye*. Online. HTTP: <https://theconversation.com/after-the-plague-shakespeare-imagined-a-world-saved-from-poison-slander-and-the-evil-eye-134608> (accessed 5 November 2020).

1 Play for health

A journey for life

Once upon a time there were just two certainties in life: that we are born and that we will die. Now, when we think about what happens on the journey between these two landmarks, we can confidently make two further assumptions. The first is that personal experiences at the start of life will have an influence on every aspect of our subsequent development (Cozolino 2006; Narvaez 2018); the second, that our subsequent development follows an indeterminate course and that there is always the potential for change and for growth (Doidge 2008, 2015).

A relational approach to health and wellbeing (Lerner 1998) emphasizes the dynamic, interactive relationship between individual development and the impact of the changing contexts of our lives (Santrock 2007). Our personal play history is one feature of this dynamic process and, in this book, we explore how the experience of play throughout the life course, sculpts and resculpts the shape of our lives: our physical health, our mental wellbeing, and our connections to the people around us and to the world in which we live. The idea of play as integral to health and development is now well supported by evidence from play theory (Pellegrini 2009), from neuroscience (Kestley 2014), and from the stories of real people playing in the real world (Leichter-Saxby 2014).

In his book, *Finite and Infinite Games*, Carse (1987: 37) asserts, 'only that which can change can continue'. The story of our playing, throughout the changing contexts of our lives, contains important clues to our lifelong health and wellbeing and therefore merits attention equal to that given to biological, social, economic, and environmental variables. A relational approach to play invites consideration of the impact of temporal and contextual change on how and what we play and of the relationship between play and our health and development. Huizinga (1955) famously proposed that play interrelates with culture – indeed that play is culture – finding expression in all aspects of our living. There is now a wealth of empirical evidence that play, located in its cultural context, interrelates with all six aspects of health – physical, mental, social, emotional, spiritual, and societal (Scriven 2017) – finding expression and meaning throughout the 'Seven Ages' of life (Shakespeare 2006).

What is health?

'Hope you're well' is a phrase which eases the way into most verbal and written exchanges, and some claim it to be so clichéd a refrain as to have become redundant (Ough 2016). Yet, this everyday greeting originates in a genuine human interest and concern about the other (Keltner et al. 2010) – albeit about more than merely their physical condition.

The idea that health is more than a matter of biology is nothing new; it's origins can be found in Ancient Greece (Tountas 2009), and it is an idea which persisted until developments in science during the eighteenth century prompted the adoption of the biomedical model of health and disease on which modern healthcare is founded.

A philosophical approach to health is important because it shapes our attitudes and behaviors toward one another, and the interchange between philosophy and medicine has played a fundamental role in conceptualizing health, particularly in the Western world (Adamson 2011). In the fourth and third century BCE, a group of physicians known as the *Hippocratics* were the first to theorize that illness was a consequence of natural, rather than supernatural, forces (Lagay 2002). They identified four bodily fluids – blood, phlegm, yellow bile, and black bile – known as humors, to which they attributed the causes of illness. *Humoral medicine* defined health as a state of humoral equilibrium and disease as a consequence of an imbalance of the humors due to 'overindulgence in food or drink, too much or too little physical exertion, or changes in the so-called naturals, i.e. the uncontrollable environment and climate' (*ibid.*). This early identification of many contemporary health concerns linked complex interactions between the physical body, lifestyle, habits, and the environment, a perception which persisted for over 2000 years, until the rise of empirical science in the mid-nineteenth century (*ibid.*).

Until the mid-eighteenth century, the prevailing orthodox Christian view of the mind–body relationship was monistic: people were perceived as spiritual beings and the body and soul as a single substantial entity. This perspective prevented scientific exploration of the human body which was prohibited on religious grounds (Mehta 2011). The proposition by Rene Descartes, in 1749, that mind and body were in fact separate entities, 'demythologized' the physical body and legitimized the study of anatomy and physiology as part of medical science (*ibid.*). Mind–body dualism laid the basis for logical medical practice that was 'based upon empirical i.e. unbiased, impersonal and unsympathetic observation and measurement' (*ibid.*: 203). At the same time, the significance of the mind for an individual's experience of health was negated and 'the field of medicine, by adhering rigidly to scientific method, mislaid its subject matter and gave up its moral responsibility toward the real health concerns of human beings' (*ibid.*: 203).

In the 1940s, the French physician Georges Canguilhem (1991) rejected the prevailing distinction between 'normal' and 'abnormal' states of health, between the notions of 'well' and 'unwell'. He recognized health to be a variable concept, different for each individual and determined by their own unique set of circumstances. For Canguilhem, health was a subjective experience defined by the individual themselves according to their functional needs. He saw health in terms of the person's ability to adapt to their environment and defined the role of the doctor as a facilitator in this process of adaptation, thus anticipating the modern concept of 'personalized medicine'. An editorial review of Canguilhem's book, published in *The Lancet* in 2009, proclaims:

> The beauty of Canguilhem's definition of health – of normality – is that it includes the animate and inanimate environment, as well as the physical, mental, and social dimensions of human life. It puts the individual patient, not the [professional], in a position of self-determining authority to define his or her health needs. The [professional] becomes a partner in delivering those needs.
>
> (The Lancet 2009)

Canguilhem's thesis finds muted resonance in the World Health Organization's original 1948 definition of health as a 'state of complete physical, mental, and social well being, . . . not merely the absence of disease or infirmity' – a definition which remains part of the WHO constitution today (World Health Organization 2019). Although widely criticized for being both vague and unrealistic, this definition of health acknowledges the inherent relationship between what Callahan (1973: 77) calls 'the good of the body and the good of the self' and endorses Canguilhem's view of health as a subjective construct. It has been argued that cultural factors are so fundamental to the promotion and nurture of health that to ignore them is to deny the potential for novel and creative efforts to change things for the better (Napier et al. 2014).

A growing acknowledgment of the scale of health inequalities in recent decades has revived awareness of the social and cultural factors influencing public health and wellbeing (Marmot 2010) and resulted in a global commitment to a 'social determinants approach' to public health. In an article published in the British Medical Journal, Huber et al. (2011) propose changing the emphasis toward health as the ability to adapt and self-manage in the face of social, physical, and emotional challenge – reflecting the essence of Canguilhem's treatise. A focus on adaptation, rather than the pursuit of an ideal state, opens the way for a more creative approach to health and development which recognizes the possibilities offered by a greater appreciation of the cultural context of people's lives – including how and why people play.

What is wellbeing?

The National Health Service in the UK defines wellbeing as 'feeling good and functioning well' (Department of Health [DoH] 2014). It refers to both an individual's experience of their life (subjective wellbeing) and the comparison of personal life circumstances with social norms and values (objective wellbeing). Put simply, 'wellbeing . . . is about "how we are doing" as individuals, communities and as a nation and how sustainable this is for the future' (What

Works Centre for Wellbeing 2019). Wellbeing matters because it affects health and longevity (DoH 2014), and maintaining optimal levels of wellbeing is considered crucial for achieving an optimal quality of life (University of California Davis Campus n.d.).

The related concept of 'wellness' describes the 'active process through which people become aware of, and make choices toward, a more successful existence' (National Wellness Institute n.d.).

Wellbeing and 'being-well' are fluctuating constructs which reflect both individual and cultural priorities across temporal and cultural dimensions. The experience of pain or of sadness, for example, is different for every individual and dependent on a range of biological, social, and cultural variables (Peacock and Patel 2008). The consequences of this complex interplay between our emotions and the circumstances of our lives are vividly depicted in the Pixar Animation Studios film *Inside Out* (Pixar 2019). Taking us inside the mind of a young person, the film caricatures five of Ekman's (2007) seven universal emotions, offering an insight into the emotional turbulence of growing up and the restorative qualities of play. *Inside Out* won numerous awards (including *Best Movie for Grown Ups who Refuse to Grow Up*) and has been widely acclaimed for pointing the lens at wellbeing and for raising awareness of emotional resilience as crucial to the successful negotiation of life's transitions (Zeedyk 2015). It provides a powerful and accessible commentary on how we function emotionally and the significance of multifactorial influences, at both individual and societal levels, for optimizing our wellbeing and consequently our physical health (What Works Centre for Wellbeing 2019).

Improving wellbeing is an indicator of social progress and a key measure of both personal and societal success, which can be achieved through 'good government and charitable activity' (What Works Centre for Wellbeing 2019) and therefore registers high on the international public health agenda. The Measuring National Wellbeing Program at the UK Office for National Statistics [ONS] is responsible for collating and distributing statistical data on subjective wellbeing. The program measures wellbeing across ten broad dimensions: 'the natural environment, personal well-being, our relationships, health, what we do, where we live, personal finance, the economy, education and skills and governance' (*ibid.*). Highlighting personal wellbeing, the *Five Ways to Wellbeing* are advocated as a long-term strategy for maximizing individual wellbeing through personal connection, being active, taking notice, keeping learning, and giving of yourself (What Works Centre for Wellbeing 2017). These five ways to wellbeing are 'integral to many activities that we care about and enjoy' (*ibid.*), many of which have playful endeavors at their heart. This direct link between play and wellbeing is captured in many of the case-stories which form the main body of this book.

The meaning of play

From the infant's mirroring of the mother's gaze, to stories at bedtime; from playground games of make-believe to the risky ventures of the teenage years;

the pranks of the office clown and family banter round the dinner table; solitary gardening and social singing. From the start of life to its close, humans are motivated to pursue experiences simply because they afford them pleasure and satisfaction. These experiences we have come to call 'play'. Perry (2019) puts it simply: 'Play takes many forms, but the heart of play is pleasure'.

Walz (2010: 11) writes that 'playing is a special type of human activity – an anthropological constant', yet most attempts to determine its meaning are characterized by ambiguity and a universal acceptance that there can be no satisfactory all-encompassing definition (Turnbull and Jenvey 2004). The capacity for play is widely recognized as an innate characteristic, deriving from primordial regions of the brain (Perry et al. 2000), but its purpose, function, and value have forever been hotly debated, reflecting not only advances in scientific understanding but the sociocultural preoccupations of time and place.

Early theorists such as Groos (1976) identified play as a uniquely biological mechanism belonging exclusively to the first stage of life. They regarded play as the means by which young mammals learn and practice essential life skills, its primary function being to preserve and promote the survival of the species. This corresponds to theoretical perspectives which hold that play serves to facilitate the mastery of skills necessary for the function of adult behaviors: the sole function of play was seen as learning, and little attention was given to the context of the play (Monbiot 2017).

The 'surplus energy' theory of play, popular in the nineteenth century, also construed play as a biological mechanism but one designed to maintain the player in a state of physiological and psychological equilibrium through the release of excesses of strength or passion (Schiller 2004). The principle of play as catharsis reemerged in a different guise with the psychoanalytic theories of the early twentieth century. These framed play as the way in which children revisit 'unpleasant and excessive experiences' in order to assimilate them, recategorizing play as a therapeutic modality (Ellis 1973). The notion of play as a means of expelling undesirable qualities is in direct contrast to Patrick's (1916) relaxation theory, which proposed that play was an opportunity to restore – rather than release – energy: 'a means to reset and relax the exhausted mental and physical faculties of an individual' (Patrick 1916 cited in Groos 1976). Such is the paradoxical nature of play theory.

In the 1920s, Karl Bühler (1924) moved beyond the idea of play as either learning, catharsis, or relaxation, claiming that play is primarily an expression of 'functional pleasure' – the enjoyment to be had from the mastery of a skill or an action – and that, in early childhood, an activity or a behavior is repeated and reinforced simply by the pleasure it generates. On this basis, he defined play as 'an activity that provides functional pleasure and is maintained because of, or for the sake of, such pleasure . . . regardless of any additional reasons for performing it, or of its results' (Bühler 1924: 508). Freud (1975) had earlier rejected the idea of a link between play and pleasure because he did not think that 'the pleasure principle' could account for the 'compulsion to repeat' play behaviors which were not of themselves pleasurable. He proffered the existence of powerful instinctual drives which overruled the drive for pleasure, and which were fundamental to the child's ability to resolve inner psychological conflict, through the enactment and reenactment of primitive feelings. But both Freud and Bühler interpreted play as an internal process which operated independently of its cultural context.

The Dutch biologist and philosopher, Buytendijk (1976) was influenced by Freud's theory of drives and proposed three original drives which he believed led to play: the drive for freedom (*Befreiungstrieb*), the drive for integration (*Vereinigungstrieb*), and the drive for repetition (*Wiederholungstreib*). The difference between Buytendijk's theory of play and its precursors rests on his proposal that play arises out of an interaction between innate drives and the context within which the play takes place, thus foreshadowing subsequent debate around the dualities of nature and nurture.

The play debate consistently returns to the seminal text of Johannes Huizinga (1955). Most contemporary play scholars concur with the central tenets of his analysis that play is an expression of free will and that it represents a 'stepping-out' from everyday life into a 'temporary sphere of activity with a disposition all its own' (Huizinga 1955: 8).

It was not until the middle of the twentieth century that the value of play was linked to its pleasure-generating, rather than exclusively functional qualities (Beach 1945). Callois's (1958) comprehensive analysis of the playing of games expanded Huizinga's definition to incorporate the notion that play is always associated with the feelings of pleasure it generates, stating: 'the player devotes himself spontaneously to the game, of his free will and for his pleasure' (Callois 1958: 6). In more recent times, Csikszentmihalyi (1981) has reemphasized the significance of 'subjective experience', reinforcing the view that it is the pleasure derived from play which both engages the player and encourages repetition of the play behavior. The importance of feelings and sensations, of the player's subjective experience of play, is now validated by neuroscientific research which has transformed our understanding of play in recent decades (Panksepp 2008).

Play and the brain

Perry et al. (2000) offer a neurodevelopmental perspective of the connection between pleasure and play. They have shown how play evolves in complexity throughout the course of our lives and how it is the pleasure associated with the play experience that drives its repetition (Figure 1.1). Perry et al. (2000: 9) write: 'The brain grows to become a dynamic ever-changing biological system which gives us the capacity to love, create, communicate or think . . . [it] becomes a product of our genetic potential and our history of experience'.

The pleasure center of the brain has been located in the *nucleus accumbens*, part of the limbic system which is responsible for controlling many aspects of human behavior. The role of the *nucleus accumbens* is to integrate motivation and action in order to trigger sensations of satisfaction and pleasure. When we

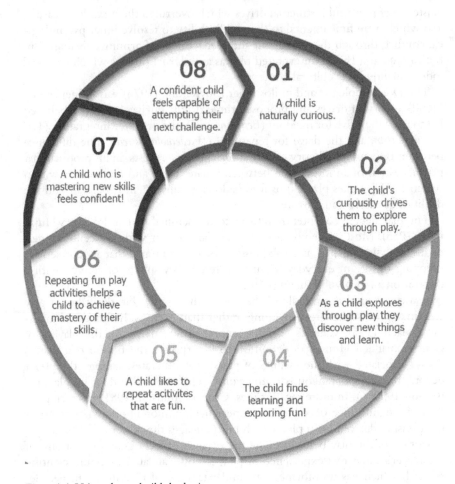

08
A confident child feels capable of attempting their next challenge.

01
A child is naturally curious.

07
A child who is mastering new skills feels confident!

02
The child's curiousity drives them to explore through play.

06
Repeating fun play activities helps a child to achieve mastery of their skills.

03
As a child explores through play they discover new things and learn.

05
A child likes to repeat acitivites that are fun.

04
The child finds learning and exploring fun!

Figure 1.1 Using play to build the brain

Source: (Gooey Brains 2016) reproduced by kind permission of Gooey Brains.

engage with pleasurable pursuits, whether they be primal drives such as eating and reproduction, or more nuanced behaviors such as play and learning, the brain releases a range of neurotransmitters, the most notable of which is the chemical dopamine. This 'feel good' hormone is regarded as fundamental to how humans negotiate their way through life, through its role in motivational salience – the prompting or repressing of specific behaviors (Puglisi-Allegra and Ventura 2012). However, the subjective experience of pleasure linked with play is not merely the outcome of a sequence of neurological processes. The wonder of the human brain is that, while it is a product of evolution, it is not sculpted solely by nature but is developed uniquely in each individual by their experience of living in the world. The wiring of the brain is not fixed at birth, or even at the end of childhood, but changes over time and with experience according to the principles of *neuroplasticity* (Doidge 2008), and play is one of the potentially transformative agents of this change. Oliker (2015) explains that 'throughout the lifespan, play supports neurological growth and development while building complex, skilled, flexible, responsive and socially adept brains'.

In her book, *How Emotions Are Made*, Lisa Feldman-Barrett (2017) makes the powerful case that each brain is wired to its unique social and physical surroundings. It follows that the pleasure derived from play is not located in the play experience itself, but in our relationship to it. This concept of *affective realism* helps to explain variations in what different individuals and societies regard as play, and how these perceptions change over time. Contemporary research with children reinforces the role of emotional pleasure as key to differentiating play from other behaviors or activities: children regard play as something they do because they want to, a voluntary activity of free will (Howard et al. 2004).

Recognition that the subjective experience of the player is central to the identification of an activity or experience as play 'underlines the humanity of play' (Walz 2010) and invites a participatory approach to an exploration of the nature of play in its sociocultural context.

Play and playfulness

The association of play with pleasure is not without criticism. Vygotsky (1933) pointed out that there are many nonplay activities which generate greater feelings of pleasure than play (most obviously related to food and sex) and that some activities identified as play (aggressive sports or certain games, for example) are not necessarily pleasurable for the player. Difficulties arise because of the conflation of the terms 'pleasure' and 'enjoyment' or 'fun' in relation to play (Blythe and Hassenzahl 2003). In *Flow: The Psychology of Happiness*, Csikszentmihalyi (1992) makes a distinction between pleasure, which he describes as the feeling of contentment experienced whenever we feel that 'expectations set by biological programs or by social conditioning have been met' (*ibid.*: 45), and enjoyment, which he associates with a sense of personal accomplishment. Both definitions acknowledge that pleasure and enjoyment are subjective experiences and, to a large extent, context specific. Blythe and Hassenzahl (2003) note that pleasure is connoted in terms of absorption, whereas 'fun' is culturally and experientially identified as a form of distraction. However, in the context of play, pleasure is used not only to describe absorption in activity but also to denote the feeling of enjoyment associated with the pleasurable experience and the motivation to repeat it.

A distinction is required here between play and the related concept of 'playfulness': while there is an overlap between the two, they are not equivalent. Bateson (2014) helpfully differentiates between 'play' and 'playful play', describing the latter as a positive disposition characterized by spontaneity and flexibility. He suggests that, while not always directly observable, playful play 'may be inferred from the context in which it occurs' (*ibid.*: 100). While 'play' refers to a broad range of self-motivated behaviors which are personally rewarding and which 'feel good' (including the 'deep play' of art and ritual), 'playfulness' typically refers to the application of a lighthearted disposition and a spontaneous willingness or inclination to deviate from social expectation so as to positively transform the meaning of an activity or a situation (Tonkin and Whitaker 2019).

Proyer et al. (2018) build on Barnett's (2007) definition of playfulness as representing the ability 'to frame or reframe everyday situations in such a way that they [are] experience[d] as entertaining, intellectually stimulating, or personally interesting'. Having a playful attitude is typically associated with creativity, including the capacity to view a serious situation from a new perspective and can facilitate coping in adverse circumstances. Proyer (2013) has shown that playful adults enjoy an active way of life, reporting greater physical and psychological health and a corresponding greater sense of life satisfaction, while Magnusen and Barnett (2013) have demonstrated that 'playfulness serves a strong adaptive function'. The value of playfulness seems to reside in its potential to 'generate novel solutions to challenges set by the social and physical environment' (Bateson 2014: 99), and, in doing so, to promote positive change with significant implications for health and development.

Play for health

In *The Ambiguity of Play*, Sutton-Smith (1997) transported the definition of play beyond biological, semantic, and aesthetic considerations, contending that 'practically anything can become an agency for some kind of play' (Sutton-Smith 1997: 6). His seven 'rhetorics' of play encompass experiences which range from the absorbing to the distracting, from extreme fun to profound seriousness. *The Ambiguity of Play* made plain that there is not something inherent in an action or experience which labels it as play, but rather that it is the context within which it occurs, and the meaning attributed to it by the player, which defines it as such. An important consideration in any attempt to understand the relationship between play, health, and development is Sutton-Smith's insistence that play is not just pleasurable for its own sake and that its true value rests in its viability, in the way in which the pleasure experienced through play transfers to our feelings about the rest of our lives and 'makes it possible to live more fully in the world, no matter how boring or painful or even dangerous ordinary reality might seem' (Sutton-Smith 2008: 95).

Sutton-Smith calls play a 'fortification' (Sutton-Smith 2008: 116) against the harsh realities of life, and contemporary research into adverse childhood experiences shows how play serves not only as a protective buffer against life's hardships but as a way of helping people to bounce back from adversity and go on to thrive (e.g., Pearson et al. 2017). A relational approach to play and health, which recognizes the significance of the interaction between biological and contextual changes throughout the life course, illustrates how 'play lets us exercise physical or mental or social adaptations that translate – directly or indirectly – into ordinary life adjustments' (Sutton-Smith 2008: 116). In a rapidly evolving world in which technology has created living and working conditions that did not exist 20 years ago (Zosh et al. 2017), the role of play as an adaptive facilitator will be crucial not only to the health and wellbeing of individuals but also to communities and to society as a whole.

Conclusion

Play is a catalyst for exploration, interaction, and resolution, an enabler that promotes a deeper awareness of the self and a richer engagement with the Other. It helps build and maintain relationships in the most unlikely and improbable circumstances. Play and playfulness are inherent in some of the most intimate and vulnerable moments of our lives, from the miracle of conception to the ritual farewells at the end of life's journey. Emotions such as joy, happiness, fear, and sadness are essential for healthy adaptation to our constantly changing circumstances and environments, and it is in our play that these emotions find authentic expression. Play and playfulness are serious fun, self-reinforcing through their impact on the pleasure circuits of the brain. This alone provides sufficient rationale for the pursuit of play for its own sake, but it is the potential for play and playfulness to contribute to the health and wellbeing of individuals and of society that further elevates its importance. As Goldstein (2012: 3) suggests: 'People would not devote so much of their lives to entertaining and enjoying themselves if these did not serve some greater purpose beyond their intrinsic merits'.

References

Adamson, P. (2011) *Health: The History of a Concept*. Online. HTTP: <www.oxford-new-histories.com/wp-content/uploads/2011/11/Health-proposal.pdf> (accessed 14 August 2019).

Barnett, L. A. (2007) The nature of playfulness in young adults. *Personality and Individual Differences*, 43: 949–958.

Bateson, P. (2014) Play, playfulness, creativity and innovation. *Animal Behavior and Cognition*, 1 (2): 99–112.

Beach, F. A. (1945) Current concepts of play in animals. *American Naturalist*, 79: 523–541.

Blythe, M. A. and Hassenzahl, M. (2003) The semantics of fun: Differentiating enjoyable experiences. In: Blythe, M. A., Overbeeke, K., Monk, A. F. and Wright, P. C. (Eds.), *Funology: From Usability to Enjoyment*. Dordrecht, the Netherlands: Kluwer Academic Publishers: 91–100.

Bühler, K. (1924) *Die geistige Entwicklung des Kindes* [Mental Development of Children]. 4th ed. Jena: Fischer.

Buytendijk, F. J. J. (1976) *Studies in Play and Games*. New York: Arno Press.

Callahan, D. (1973) The WHO definition of health. *The Hastings Center Studies*, 1 (3): 77–87.

Callois, R. (1958) *Man, Play and Games*. Online. HTTP: <http://voidnetwork.gr/wp-content/uploads/2016/09/Man-Play-and-Games-by-Roger-Caillois.pdf> (accessed 15 May 2019).

Canguilhem, G. (1991) *The Normal and the Pathological*. New York: Zone Books.

Carse, J. (1987) *Finite and Infinite Games: A Vision of Life as Play and Possibility*. New York: Ballantine Books.

Cozolino, L. (2006) *The Neuroscience of Human Relationships: Attachment and the Developing Social Brain*. New York: W. W. Norton & Co.

Csikszentmihalyi, M. (1981) Some paradoxes in the definition of play. In: Cheska, A. (Ed.), *Play as Context: 1979 Proceedings of the Association for the Anthropological Study of Play*. West Point, NY: Leisure Press: 14–26.

Csikszentmihalyi, M. (1992) *Flow: The Psychology of Happiness*. London: Rider, Random House.

Department of Health (2014) *Wellbeing: Why It Matters to Health Policy*. Online. HTTP: <http://assets.publishing.service.gov.uk/government/uploads/system/uploads/attachment_data/file/277566/Narrative__January_2014_.pdf>

Doidge, N. (2008) *The Brain That Changes Itself*. London: Penguin.

Doidge, N. (2015) *The Brain's Way of Healing: Remarkable Discoveries and Recoveries from the Frontiers of Neuroplasticity*. London: Penguin.

Ekman, P. (2007) *Emotions Revealed: Recognizing Faces and Feelings to Improve Communication and Emotional Life*. New York: Holt Paperbacks.

Ellis, M. J. (1973) *Why People Play*. Englewood Cliffs, NJ: Prentice-Hall.

Feldman-Barrett, L. (2017) *How Emotions Are Made*. London: Pan Macmillan.

Freud, S. (1975) *Beyond the Pleasure Principle*. New York: Norton.

Goldstein, J. (2012) *Play in Children's Development, Health and Wellbeing*. Brussels: Toy Industries of Europe.

Gooey Brains (2016) *Using Play to Build the Brain*. Online. HTTP: <https://gooeybrains.com/2016/04/10/using-play-to-build-the-brain/> (accessed 26 August 2019).

Groos, K. (1976) *The Play of Animals*. New York: Arno Press.

Howard, J., Jenvey, V. and Hill, C. (2004) Children's categorization of play and learning based on social context. *Early Child Development and Care*, 176 (3/4): 379–393.

Huber, M., Knottnerus, J. A., Green, L., van der Horst, H., Jadad, A., Kromhout, D. (. . .) and Smid, H. (2011) How should we define health? *British Medical Journal*, 343: d4163.

Huizinga, J. (1955) *Homo Ludens: A Study of the Play-Element in Culture*. Boston, MA: Beacon Press.

Keltner, K., Marsh, J. and Smith, J. A. (2010) *The Compassionate Instinct: The Science of Human Goodness*. New York: W.W. Norton and Co.

Kestley, T. A. (2014) *The Interpersonal Neurobiology of Play: Brain-Building Interventions for Emotional Well-Being*. New York: W.W. Norton and Co.

Lagay, F. (2002) *The Legacy of Humoral Medicine*. Online. HTTP: <https://journalofethics.ama-assn.org/article/legacy-humoral-medicine/2002-07> (accessed 6 July 2019).

The Lancet (2009) Editorial: What is health? The ability to adapt. *The Lancet*, 373 (9666): 781.

Leichter-Saxby, M. (2014) Memories of and reflections on play. *International Journal of Play*, 3 (1): 6–8.

Lerner, R. M. (1998) Theories of human development: Contemporary perspectives. In: Lerner, R. M. (Ed.), *Handbook of Child Psychology: Theoretical Models of Human Development*. Vol. 1, 5th ed. New York: John Wiley & Sons: 1–24.

Magnusen, C. D. and Barnett, L. A. (2013) The playful advantage: How playfulness enhances coping with stress. *Leisure Sciences*, 35 (2): 129–144.

Marmot, M. (2010) *Fair Society Healthy Lives (Full Report)*. London: The Marmot Review.

Mehta, N. (2011) Mind-body dualism: A critique from a health perspective. *Mens Sana Monographs*, 9 (1): 202–209. doi:10.4103/0973-1229.77436.

Monbiot, G. (2017, 15 February) In an age of robots, schools are teaching our children to be redundant. *The Guardian*. Online. HTTP: <www.theguardian.com/commentisfree/2017/feb/15/robots-schools-teaching-children-redundant-testing-learn-future> (accessed 14 August 2019).

Napier, A. D., Ancarno, C., Butler, B., Calabreses, J., Chater, A., Chatterjee, H. [. . .] and Woolf, K. (2014) Culture and health. *Lancet*, 384: 1607–1639. doi:10.1016/S0140-6736 (14)61603-2.

Narvaez, D. (2018) *Basic Needs, Wellbeing and Morality: Fulfilling Human Potential*. London: Palgrave Pivot–Palgrave Macmillan.

National Wellness Institute (n.d.) *About Wellness*. Online. HTTP: <htttp://nationalwellness. org/page/AboutWellness> (accessed 21 August 2019).

Oliker, D. M. (2015) *Let's Play: How the Science of the Brain Is Changing Therapy: The Increasing Importance of Play, Creativity and Spontaneity*. Online. HTTP: <www.psychologytoday. com/intl/blog/the-long-reach-childhood/201504/let-s-play-how-the-science-the-brain-is-changing-therapy?amp> (accessed 2 May 2019).

Ough, T. (2016) *Stop Writing 'I Hope You're Well' in Emails: Here's What to Say Instead*. Online. HTTP: <www.telegraph.co.uk/education-and-careers/0/you-need-to-stop-writing-i-hope-youre-well-in-emails-heres-wha/> (accessed 12 August 2019).

Panksepp, J. (2008) Play, ADHD, and the construction of the social brain. *American Journal of Play* Summer: 55–79.

Patrick, G. T. W. (1916) *The Psychology of Relaxation*. Houghton, NY: Mifflin.

Peacock, S. and Patel, S. (2008) Cultural influences on pain. *Reviews in Pain*, 1 (2): 6–9.

Pearson, E., Umayahara, M. and Ndijuye, L. (2017) *Play and Resilience*. Online. HTTP: <https://docplayer.net/86520958-Supporting-childhood-resilience-through-play-a-facilitation-guide-for-early-childhood-practitioners.html> (accessed 17 January 2021).

Pellegrini, A. (2009) *The Role of Play in Human Development*. Oxford: Oxford University Press.

Perry, B. D. (2019) *Emotional Development: The Importance of Pleasure in Play*. Online. HTTP: <www.scholastic.com/teachers/articles/teaching-content/emotional-development-importance-pleasure-play/> (accessed 26 March 2019).

Perry, B. D., Hogan, L. and Marlin, S. J. (2000) Curiosity, pleasure and play: A neurodevelopmental perspective. *Haaeyc Advocate*, August: 9–12.

Pixar (2019) *Disney Pixar Inside Out*. Online. HTTP: <www.pixar.com/feature-films/inside-out> (accessed 13 August 2019).

Proyer, R. T. (2013) The well-being of playful adults: Adult playfulness, subjective well-being, physical well-being, and the pursuit of enjoyable activities. *European Journal of Humour Research*, 1 (1): 84–98.

Proyer, R. T., Gander, F., Bertenshaw, E. J. and Brauer, K. (2018) The positive relationships of playfulness with indicators of health, activity and physical fitness. *Frontiers in Psychology*, 9: 1440.

Puglisi-Allegra, S. and Ventura, R. (2012) Prefrontal/accumbal catecholamine system processes high motivational salience. *Frontiers in Behavioral Neuroscience*, 6: 31.

Santrock, J. W. (2007) *A Topical Approach to Life-Span Development*. New York: McGraw-Hill.

Schiller, F. (2004) *On the Aesthetic Education of Man*. New York: Dover Books on Western Philosophy.

Scriven, A. (2017) *Ewles & Simnett's Promoting Health: A Practical Guide*. 7th ed. London: Elsevier.

Shakespeare, W. (2006) *As You Like It*. London: The Arden Shakespeare, Third Series.

Sutton-Smith, B. (1997) *The Ambiguity of Play*. Cambridge, MA: Harvard University Press.

Sutton-Smith, B. (2008) Play theory: A personal journey and new thoughts. *American Journal of Play*: 80–123.

Tonkin, A. and Whitaker, J. (Eds.) (2019) *Play and Playfulness for Public Health and Wellbeing*. London: Routledge.

Tountas, Y. (2009) The historical origins of the basic concepts of health promotion and education: The role of ancient Greek philosophy and medicine. *Health Promotion International*, 24 (2): 185–192. doi:10.1093/heapro/dap006.

Turnbull, J. and Jenvey, V. B. (2004) Criteria used by adults and children to categorize subtypes of play. *Early Child Development and Care*, 176 (5): 539–551.

University of California Davis Campus (n.d.) *What Is Wellness*. Online. HTTP: <https://shcs.ucdavis.edu/wellness/what-is-wellness> (accessed 6 July 2019).

Vygotsky, L. (1933) *Play and Its Role in the Mental Development of the Child*. Online. HTTP: <www.marxists.org/archive/vygotsky/works/1933/play.htm> (accessed 9 May 2019).

Walz, S. P. (2010) *Toward a Ludic Architecture: The Space of Play and Games*. London: ETC Press.

What Works Centre for Wellbeing (2017) *Five Ways to Wellbeing in the UK*. Online. HTTP: <https://whatworkswellbeing.org/blog/five-ways-to-wellbeing-in-the-uk/> (accessed 13 August 2019).

What Works Centre for Wellbeing (2019) *What Is wellbeing?* Online. HTTP: <https://whatworkswellbeing.org/about/what-is-wellbeing/> (accessed 12 August 2019).

World Health Organization (2019) *Constitution*. Online. HTTP: <www.who.int/about/who-we-are/constitution> (accessed 12 August 2019).

Zeedyk, S. (2015) *Pixar's 'Inside Out': A Lesson in Loss*. Online. HTTP: <http://suzannezeedyk.co.uk/wp2/tag/inside-out/> (accessed 21 August 2019).

Zosh, J., Hopkins, E., Jensen, H., Liu, C., Neale, D., Hirsh-Pasek, K., Solis, S. and Whitebread, D. (2017) *Learning through Play: A Review of the Evidence (White Paper)*. Denmark: The Lego Foundation.

2 Tell me a story

Stories have been used since the beginning of time not only to recount the details of an experience or event, to engage, and to entertain but also to convey messages or themes of serious importance, messages that might influence the listeners' health, wellbeing, or even their very survival. Using stories to communicate the value of play for lifelong health and wellbeing represents the adoption of this age-old narrative tradition; taking a narrative approach to professional practice shares common features with our day-to-day storytelling, in that it 'incorporate[s] temporality, a social context, complicating events, and an evaluative conclusion that together make a coherent story' (McAlpine 2016).

The 'case-stories' featured in this book not only illustrate the transformative potential of play-based experience but also have the power to challenge existing perceptions and attitudes to play and to motivate action, and they can be a valuable way of engaging others with quality improvement work (The Health Foundation 2016). Clare Patey, director of Empathy Museum (n.d.), is quoted as saying, 'Stories have a transformative power to allow us to see the world in a different way than we do if we just encounter it on our own', they represent 'an opportunity to learn from another person's experience [which] can shape, strengthen or challenge our [own] opinions and values' (cited in The Health Foundation 2016). The author Jeanette Winterson (2011: 61) elucidates: 'Personal stories work for other people when those stories become both paradigms and parables. The intensity of a story . . . releases it into a bigger space than the one it occupied in time and place'.

From symbolic communication to a narrative approach

Humans are the most sociable of all primates (Radford 2019): we have been described as the 'mammalian bee' (Monbiot 2014), sharing with bees a complex sociality – a trait which originated as an evolutionary survival response (Public Library of Science 2016). Social survival depends on finding common ways of communicating messages of collective importance, and social evolution demands that these messages allow for the possibility of novelty and change.

Symbolic communication – the use of a shared representational system to communicate meaning – is recognized as a crucial step in the social evolution of *Homo sapiens*, facilitating cultural evolution and the emergence of human language (Grouchy et al. 2016). There is a common assumption that humans are the only species that possess natural symbolic communication systems, but the 'dance communication' of the honeybee suggests otherwise (Barron and Aino Plath 2017). The honeybee dance is a unique form of animal signaling which involves the use of movement and social interaction as meaningful communication. In a remarkable demonstration of cooperative behavior, honeybees dance to indicate the location of valuable resources to their nestmates and to recruit additional foragers to those resources (*ibid.*). Like humans, honeybees have evolved to share meaningful 'stories' as a matter of both physical and social survival.

Symbolic communication requires that all parties to an interaction attribute reciprocal meaning to a system of symbols (actions, images, objects). Langsdorf (2017) cites the Changing Minds organization: 'Symbols are communications that have specific meaning. Usually visual, symbols act as communication short-cuts that convey one or more messages that have been previously learned by both the sender and the recipient'. The effectiveness of the honeybee dance depends on all the 'dancers' sharing a common understanding of its component features. It follows that the use of symbolic communication can be understood as a 'short cut to the brain' (*ibid.*) enabling complex ideas to be transmitted in 'the blink of an eye' or, in the case of the bees, an abdominal 'waggle' (Barron and Aino Plath 2017).

Symbolic communication is the starting point for the complex communication systems which make up human language (Grouchy et al. 2016), and it is this evolutionary adaptation which has enabled humans to become 'story telling animals . . . [through the] transmission of skills and knowledge as fable, epic or cautionary tale' (Radford 2019). Playing with words 'until they can impersonate physical objects and abstract ideas' (Ackerman cited in Popova 2016) allows for the representation of a message in differing formats and presentation styles (Storytelling Brands 2019). The sharing of stories takes many different forms, including visual art, dance, and dramatic performance – as well as the spoken and written word – and throughout human history, stories have been used, like the dance communication of the honeybee, to transmit knowledge and ideas which challenge *a priori* expectations.

A brief history of storytelling for personal development and social change

The first representation of influential storytelling is believed to be the Chauvet cave paintings in South-west France which have been dated at between 30,000 and 32,000 years old. While the meaning behind the cave paintings – which depict 14 animal species, as well as abstract forms – remains ambiguous, it has been speculated that they tell the story of a volcanic eruption in the area and were possibly intended as a warning against future danger (Callaway 2016).

In Ancient Greece, storytellers were highly esteemed members of society and were generously rewarded for their epic tales. Sloan (2018) describes how the humanistic quality of these ancient myths and legends served to transform them from lyrical poetry to become 'the vehicle that catalyzed profound individual, cultural and political change'. Stories united the ancient Greeks with a common language and moral code and a collective identity. The famous fables of Aesop (620 BCE –564 BCE), for example, deliver valuable lessons in how to live as part of a cohesive social group; initially addressed to adults on religious, social, and political themes, *Aesop's Fables* represents possibly the earliest form of social-skills training. The Greek author Philostratus wrote of Aesop: 'like those who dine well off the plainest dishes, he made use of humble incidents to teach great truths' (Livius.org 2019). The various case-stories which make up the main body of this book have been collated and shared in an attempt to impart the 'great truth' that play – in all its forms – is essential to our health and wellbeing.

The most widely published storybook of all time is The Bible, with an estimated five billion copies sold and distributed worldwide (Guinness World Records 2019). Like the myths and legends of earlier times, the stories of the Old Testament and the New Testament represent a series of lessons for life, using metaphor to address the fundamental questions of the human condition. The historical authority of the Bible is based on the tenet that it was written by the principal players in the events described, which both affords it credibility and may account for its broad appeal and influence. This provenance has been robustly denied, but underlying it is the fact that personal narrative has a unique potency.

The social impact of personal narrative is reflected in contemporary recognition of the value of storytelling for the promotion of positive health. Freire and Macedo (1987) contend that the first act of personal agency is 'speaking the world': being able to use one's own words to describe personal experiences, in the safe knowledge that they will be listened to and respected by an audience. Labonte et al. (1999: 40) expand this idea, proposing that 'as stories are shared between people, they become "generative themes" for group reflection, analysis and action planning', a concept examined in more detail later in this chapter.

William Shakespeare (1564–1614), perhaps the greatest ever playwright in the English language, was a master storyteller. His opus of 37 plays revolves around four universal themes or motifs – conflict, appearance and reality, order and disorder, and change (Gibson 2016). Like the Bible, Shakespeare's plays 'speak the world' (Freire and Macedo 1987) because these themes engage the audience in a personal relationship with the story. Shakespeare created complex, evolving inner lives for his characters which underlie their relatability to audiences across different historical and cultural contexts (No Sweat Shakespeare 2019a). Hamlet's grief at the loss of his father and resentment of his mother's swift recoupling are as recognizable to the modern audience as they would have been 400 years ago. The gender conflicts in *Much Ado About Nothing* and the graphic portrayal of mental illness in *King Lear* are as relevant today as they were at the time of writing.

In the second act of *As You Like It*, one of Shakespeare's most popular and oft-adapted comedies, the character Jacques delivers the famous monologue which has come to be known as 'The Seven Ages of Man' and which served as the inspiration for this book. Shakespeare likens the world to a stage on which 'all the men and women [are] merely players', offering a caricature of each of the stages of life in a humorous yet profound portrayal of lifespan development. Shakespeare was not alone in taking a lifespan approach to human development – Hippocrates also recognized seven life stages (Aristotle only three) – and the number seven features widely in philosophical and religious theory (No Sweat Shakespeare 2019b). In *As You Like It*, 'gender roles, nature and politics are confused in a play that reflects on how bewildering yet utterly pleasurable life can be' (Royal Shakespeare Company 2019) – a complex interplay of themes which recur throughout the literary canon.

Comparable themes relating to family, society, and personal and social development are found in the symbolic archetypes of the popular fairytales of the nineteenth century, such as those of the Brothers Grimm and Hans Christian Andersen. These folk stories and fairytales are thought to have their roots in a common cultural history dating back to the birth of the Indo-European languages. However, Dr Jamie Tehrani, anthropologist at Durham University, has found that 'some of these stories go back much further than the earliest literary records and indeed further back than Classical mythology' (BBC 2019a) reinforcing the idea that stories have always been used to engage people with matters of profound importance.

Booker (2004) has identified seven common narrative themes in the social history of storytelling. This commonality is no coincidence because the themes embodied in stories, both ancient and modern, reflect basic human needs and desires and allow for the exploration of shared human impulses, thoughts, fears, and aspirations (Hefferman 2017). Kennedy (cited in Storlie 2014) suggests that a great story is one that symbolizes a human challenge or condition that calls for bravery, or the overcoming of a conflict of values, which the listener or reader can identify with or apply to their own lives.

Walters (2017: 56) writes: 'Fairytales and folktales are part of the cultural conserve that can be used to address children's fears . . . and give them some role training in an approach that honors the children's window of tolerance'. The case-story, used in the context of health and wellbeing, follows this custom of presenting a profound and psychologically challenging theme in a manageable format which 'honors the window of [our] tolerance' (*ibid.*). It illustrates a complex theoretical perspective in condensed form, allowing for an in-depth understanding of the topic and a credible platform from which to launch further investigation of the theme.

The use of narrative for knowledge development

Capturing evidence of efficacy within the fields of health and the social sciences does not always lend itself to the conventional, positivist approaches derived from quantitative research paradigms (Labonte et al. 1999). While efficacy is important, especially in times of austerity (Hannah 2014), it is people who make practice, and practitioners in health and social care have long advocated for a more constructivist approach to gathering evidence which is better suited to capturing the essence of their practice (Morgan 2012). The rise of the 'expert patient' and the proliferation of first-person accounts of health-care experiences from both sides of the patient–professional divide (e.g., Engelberg 2014; Kay 2018) make a strong case for the role of storytelling as a route to greater understanding and to more creative intervention based on empathy and a desire for reciprocity in the helping relationship. It is helpful here to note Paley and Eva's (2005) differentiation of storytelling from the more conventional use of narrative in healthcare. They define *narrative* as 'the sequence of events and the (claimed) causal connections between them' and *story* as 'an interweaving of plot and character, whose organization is designed to elicit a certain emotional response from the reader'. It is the emotional element of storytelling which engages us in a process of reflection, prompting action for change and personal growth.

The concept of reflectiveness *in practice* (thinking while doing) and *on practice* (after the event) was popularized by Donald Schon in his seminal text, *The reflective practitioner: how professionals think in action*, published in 1983 (Finlay 2008). In counterpoint to the established knowledge-based model of professional practice, Schon (1991, cited in Hargreaves and Page 2013: 164) proposed that the 'practice of a profession is where learning should start, with application and theory following from this'. When fledgling professionals discuss their experiences of practice, it is often through the recounting of events, the sharing of anecdotes (stories), and the venting of emotion that learning takes place. Hargreaves and Page (2013: 11) explain: 'Storytelling is something that all people do – we use stories to explain, construct and understand our lives. Reflective practice often revolves around story telling'.

Storytelling is a powerful medium for reflective practice in the health and social sciences in that it represents the narration of factual events in a context which also allows for the safe expression and exploration of feelings, values, and beliefs. However, Morgan (2012) reminds us that 'stories are powerful because they show people as human beings and their emotions, so they need to be handled very sensitively'. Paley and Eva (2005: 83) advise 'narrative vigilance' due to the emotional persuasiveness of some stories over others. Knowing that reflective stories package essential truths within a fictional context is a reminder that a narrative account can never be a substitute for actual experience (Hargreaves and Page 2013: 13). The ethical practice of health and social care demands that the process of how care is delivered is just as important as the outcome of that care which implies a readiness on the part of the practitioner to acknowledge their emotionality (Hargreaves and Page 2013). Public inquiries into adverse healthcare incidents have repeatedly highlighted the role of culture in the delivery of care and emphasized the need to overcome the cultural barriers to change and improvement which derive from unacknowledged preconceptions (Tonkin and Whitaker 2016).

Systems theory recognizes that the course of individual development is influenced by an amalgamation of the experiences, events, and transitions that occur during the course of a lifetime (Bronfenbrenner 2009). The stories of our lives are similarly transformed as we move through the lifespan. Just as the details of a story change with each remembering and retelling, so its interpretation is transformed by time and circumstance. Henderson (2018) endorses the view that the act of sharing a personal story inevitably situates the teller within a particular sociocultural context and that 'the activity of writing itself filters the world through the lens of the writer, a personal analysis of life events' (*ibid.*: 104). Storytelling is always a collaborative interaction between the teller and the listener; Langer (2016) argues that listening and giving attention is perhaps the most basic and powerful way to connect with others.

From social narrative to a 'case-story' approach

Stories are the basic ingredients of social communication: it has been estimated that as much as 65 per cent of all human interaction takes the form of social storytelling (Hefferman 2017). Research in the field of neuroscience now demonstrates that storytelling engages the psychological processes needed to gain access to the subjective experience of others, which is 'a crucial skill that enables the complex social relationships that characterize human societies' (Kid and Castano 2013). Stories connect us to the past and to each other and act as a gateway to the future, prompting Westenberg (2017) to declare that 'storytelling is the greatest technology that humans have ever created'.

In acknowledgment of the oral traditions of local communities and the impact of women's personal stories for the modern feminist movement, Labonte et al. (1999) propose a 'story/dialogue' approach to knowledge development in health education in response to practitioner concerns that a conventional, positivist methodology is inadequate for understanding and evaluating health promotion pedagogy. In a subversion of the maxim, 'there's nothing so practical as a good theory' (Lewin 1943), they assert that 'there's nothing so theoretical as a good practice' and advocate for the use of 'case stories' as 'a grounding base against which probing questions can be asked about what was done, why it was done and what it accomplished' (Labonte et al. 1999: 40). A case-story approach has come to represent an adjunct to other qualitative research methods used in the health and social sciences, recognizing that 'we continually create and refine our experience, and indeed our moral agency, through the stories that we tell' (Gunaratnam n.d.)

In the research by Labonte et al. (1999), participants were invited to prepare a case-story around a so-called *generative theme*, which focused on the power relationship between participants in a practice situation, rather than the content of that practice. Dialogue around the case-story enabled practitioners to explore how tensions were dealt with in the context of what happened, and what actions were taken as a result; a synthesis of the insights gleaned from several stories allowed for more generalized learning to take place (*ibid.*).

In this book, we have borrowed the concept of the case-story to illustrate a diversity of 'play-full' approaches to health and wellbeing which have 'the quality of being well-founded on experience' (Heron 1988). Stories are not a substitute for experience in health and social care: they represent new experiences, reshaping expectations and allowing us 'to envision alternative futures' (Flyvbjerg 2006). In *Letting Stories Breathe* (2010), the sociologist Arthur Frank borrows the description of stories as our 'companion species' because they 'work with people, for people, and always stories work *on* people, affecting what people are able to see as real, as possible' (p. 3). Our case-stories do not reflect a generative theme or deploy Labonte's rigorous dialogue methodology, but they offer insights into the ways in which play and playfulness are being conceptualized in the context of personal and public health and wellbeing. Through a depiction of 'what happened through people, place and plot' (Storlie 2014) which acknowledges the emotionality of subjective experience, these case-stories invite the reader to consider the potency of the 'play-story' for both personal and professional development.

The power of storytelling

Zeig's (1980) analysis of the use of anecdotes in psychotherapy is helpful in isolating some of the key features which make the sharing of stories such a potent strategy for challenging social perceptions of play and for stimulating the exploration of playful approaches to meeting health and wellbeing priorities.

Stories are engaging

Stories 'speak to the heart' (Pelias 2004) because they first 'speak to the brain'. Research in the field of neuroscience has shown that a descriptive story triggers the sensory receptors in the neural cortex in a way that a factual text does not. Stories seem to light up the same parts of the brain that are active when we actually experience something, creating a simulation of reality (Schwertly 2014). When we read or listen to a story, we tend to relate it to our own experience: the insular cortex of the brain seeks out an emotionally relevant context for our sensory response to the story which then triggers feelings of empathy and compassion. Jennifer Aakar (cited in Schwertly 2014) is quoted as saying:

> Research shows our brains are not hard-wired to understand logic or retain facts for very long. Our brains are wired to understand and retain stories. A story is a journey that moves the listener and when the listener goes on that journey, they feel different and the result is persuasion and sometimes action.

Stories are non-threatening

'Story doctor', Susan Perrow (2012: 11), writing about the use of metaphor in storytelling, explains that stories 'speak directly to the imagination, building connections through feeling rather than theory or abstract reasoning' and are thus effective ways of addressing difficult or challenging themes. Stories reach the unconscious mind in a discreet and subtle way, which allows the reader or listener to accept and absorb their meaning in a manner that's both different from, and more impactful than, listening to the same message delivered more directly.

Stories speak to the individual and therefore foster independence of thought and action

Each person reading or listening to a story will respond to its theme in a personal way in relation to their own interests and experiences and will then arrive at their own unique conclusion or self-initiated action. The curiosity aroused by a story leads the reader or listener to search inside themselves for resources to make sense of the theme and to apply it to their own situation.

Stories model flexibility

Stories introduce the possibility of variations in thought and behavior by suggesting alternative interpretations of life events and by offering an insight into different opinions and behavioral choices. When we read or listen to tales of people doing something different, we must suspend our usual way of thinking about the world and accept that there are multiple ways of addressing the same issues and challenges. Hefferman (2017) identifies this as fundamental to the way in which we 'develop a better understanding of the world and those we share it with'.

Stories bypass a natural resistance to change

Humans are creatures of habit and tend to repeat familiar patterns of behavior, whether they are helpful or not: it can be difficult to veer away from the safety of tried-and-tested ways of thinking about, and being, in the world. Stories nudge the reader or listener toward new possibilities, rather than prescribing a specific course of action.

When we use stories to illustrate the links between play and health, we encourage a shift from convergent to divergent thinking. Rosen (2010: 99) writes that 'in divergent thinking, one idea moves out into many different directions, like the branching of a tree'. We can free ourselves from a limited perception of play as belonging uniquely to childhood or to our own specific domain of interest and, rather than focusing on the limitations to play, we can choose to focus on the play itself.

Stories are about a relationship

There is an old Scottish saying that a story needs to be told 'eye to eye, mind to mind and heart to heart'. A story needs an audience: a reader or a listener.

The sharing of stories involves reaching out to another in a spirit of openness and generosity – trusting the other to accept and respect the message conveyed. Martin Buber (1878–1965) teaches that it is only in relationship with other people that we can find personal fulfillment and grow as independent beings, a view reinforced by Maslow's (1943) contention that it is the need for emotional connection that drives all human behavior.

Stories are memorable

The emotional impact of a story shared and received is that it imprints itself on the memory. Information conveyed in narrative rather than factual form is 22 times more memorable (Radford 2019), making storytelling an effective (and more engaging) way of developing knowledge and understanding. Whether we remember the exact wording of a story or the character or style of the storyteller, the essence of the tale and the experience of reading or listening to it are irrevocably etched on the unconscious mind. In the words of author Phillip Pullman: '*Thou shalt not* is soon forgotten, but *Once upon a time* lasts forever' (BBC 2019b).

Conclusion

Storytelling is a defining feature of our humanity and of our desire to connect to our fellow beings. We all tell stories about ourselves and our lives every day: both to ourselves and to each other. These stories represent an ongoing attempt to organize, understand, and communicate our thoughts, feelings, and actions and, in doing so, to imbue our lives with a coherent meaning (Storr 2019).

Perhaps, the greatest value of a narrative approach to play is its potential to explore the multiple ways of 'knowing' play (Pinnegar and Daynes 2007). The use of case-stories to reinforce the links between play and health recognizes and respects 'the power of subjectivity' in opening up the conversation about play's contribution to the health agenda and in broadening the range of contributors to the play debate (Garvis 2015). The 'great truth' that play is essential to lifelong health and wellbeing can be found in all sorts of surprising places.

References

Barron, A. and Aino Plath, J. (2017) The evolution of honey bee dance communication: A mechanistic perspective. *Journal of Experimental Biology*, 220: 4339–4346. doi:10.1242/jeb.142778.

BBC (2019a) *Fairy Tale Origins Thousands of Years Old, Researchers Say*. Online. HTTP: <www.bbc.co.uk/news/uk-35358487> (accessed 3 July 2019).

BBC (2019b) *Phillip Pullman: Angels and Daemons*. Online. HTTP: <www.bbc.co.uk/programmes/b09vdpzw> (accessed 30 November 2019).

Booker, C. (2004) *The Seven Basic Plots: Why We Tell Stories*. New York: Continuum.

Bronfenbrenner, U. (2009) *The Ecology of Human Development: Experiments by Nature and Design*. Cambridge, MA: Harvard University Press.

Callaway, E. (2016) 'Cave of forgotten dreams' may hold earliest painting of volcanic eruption. *Nature*. Online. HTTP: <www.nature.com/news/cave-of-forgotten-dreams-may-hold-earliest-painting-of-volcanic-eruption-1.19177> (accessed 3 July 2019).

Empathy Museum (n.d.) *Home*. Online. HTTP: <www.empathymuseum.com/> (accessed 17 November 2020).

Engelberg, M. (2014) *Cancer Made Me a Shallower Person: A Memoir in Comics*. New York: Harper Perennial.

Finlay, L. (2008) *Reflecting on 'Reflective Practice'*. Online. HTTP: <www.open.ac.uk/opencetl/sites/www.open.ac.uk.opencetl/files/files/ecms/web-content/Finlay-(2008)-Reflecting-on-reflective-practice-PBPL-paper-52.pdf> (accessed 7 November 2019).

Flyvbjerg, B. (2006) Five misunderstandings about case-study research. *Qualitative Inquiry*, 12 (2): 219–245.

Frank, A. (2010) *Letting Stories Breathe: A Socio-Narratology*. Chicago: University of Chicago Press.

Freire, P. and Macedo, D. (1987) *Literacy: Reading the Word and the World*. South Hadley, MA: Bergin and Garvey.

Garvis, S. (2015) *Narrative Constellations: Exploring Lived Experience in Education*. Rotterdam: Sense Publishers.

Gibson, R. (2016) *Teaching Shakespeare*. Cambridge: Cambridge University Press.

Grouchy, P., D'Eleuterio, G., Christiansen, M. and Lipson, H. (2016) On the evolutionary origin of symbolic communication. *Scientific Reports*, 6: Article number 34615.

Guinness World Records Limited (2019) Online. HTTP: <www.guinnessworldrecords.com/world-records/best-selling-book-of-non-fiction/> (accessed 3 July 2019).

Gunaratnam, Y. (n.d.) *Narrative Stories*. Online. HTTP: <www.case-stories.org/narrative-ethics> (accessed 5 December 2019).

Hannah, M. (2014) *Humanizing Healthcare: Patterns of Hope for a System under Strain*. Axminster: International Futures Forum.

Hargreaves, J. and Page, L. (2013) *Reflective Practice*. Cambridge: Polity.

The Health Foundation (2016) *The Power of Storytelling*. Online. HTTP: <www.health.org.uk/newsletter-feature/power-of-storytelling> (accessed 1 July 2019).

Hefferman, M. (2017, 23 February) *The Power of Storytelling and How It Affects Your Brain*. [Blog post]. Online. HTTP: <https://talesfortadpoles.ie/blogs/news/the-power-of-storytelling-and-how-it-affects-your-brain> (accessed 26 October 2019).

Henderson, E. (2018) *Autoethnography in Early Childhood Education and Care*. Oxon: Routledge.

Heron, J. (1988) Validity in cooperative inquiry. In: Reasons, P. (Ed.), *Human Inquiry in Action*. London: Sage: 40–59.

Kay, A. (2018) *This Is Going to Hurt*. London: Picador.

Kid, D. C. and Castano, E. (2013) Reading literary fiction improves theory of mind. *Science*, 342 (6156): 377–380.

Labonte, R., Feather, J. and Hills, M. (1999) A story/dialogue method for health promotion knowledge development and evaluation. *Health Education Research*, 14 (1): 39–50.

Langer, N. (2016) The power of storytelling and the preservation of memories . . . *Educational Gerontology*, 42 (11): 739.

Langsdorf, H. (2017) *Symbols Are Shortcuts for Our Brains*. Online. HTTPS: <https://thoughtsdrawnout.com.au/symbols-are-short-cuts-for-our-brains/> (accessed 12 January 2021).

Lewin, K. (1943) Psychology and the process of group living. *Journal of Social Psychology*, 17: 113–131.

Livius.org (2019) *Philostratus, Life of Apollonius 5.11–15*. Online. HTTP: <www.livius.org/sources/content/philostratus-life-of-apollonius/philostratus-life-of-apollonius-5.11-15/> (accessed 18 June 2019).

Maslow, A. (1943) A theory of human motivation. *Psychological Review*, 50 (4): 370–396.

McAlpine, L. (2016) *Why Might You Use Narrative Methodology? A Story about Narrative*. Online. HTTP: <http://eha.ut.ee/wp-content/uploads/2016/04/6_02b_alpine.pdf> (accessed 26 June 2019).

Monbiot, G. (2014, 14 October) The age of loneliness is killing us. *The Guardian*. Online. HTTP: <www.theguardian.com/commentisfree/2014/oct/14/age-of-loneliness-killing-us> (accessed 5 November 2019).

Morgan, S. (2012, 24 April) *The Power of Story Telling*. [Blog post]. Online. HTTP: <www.health.org.uk/blogs/the-power-of-story-telling> (accessed 27 October 2019).

No Sweat Shakespeare (2019a) *Shakespeare's Play Themes*. Online. HTTP: <www.nosweatshakespeare.com/play-summary/play-themes/> (accessed 4 July 2019).

No Sweat Shakespeare (2019b) *The Seven Ages of Man*. Online. HTTP: <www.nosweatshakespeare.com/resources/seven-ages-of-man/> (accessed 27 November 2019).

Paley, J. and Eva, G. (2005) Narrative vigilance: The analysis of stories in health care. *Nursing Philosophy*, 6 (2): 83–97.

Pelias, R. J. (2004) *A Methodology of the Heart: Evoking Academic and Daily Life*. Oxford: Altamira Press.

Perrow, S. (2012) *Therapeutic Storytelling: 101 Healing Stories for Children*. Stroud: Hawthorn Press.

Pinnegar, S. and Daynes, J. G. (2007) Locating narrative inquiry historically: Thematics in the turn to narrative. In: Clandinin, D. J. (Ed.), *Handbook of Narrative Inquiry: Mapping a Methodology*. Thousand Oaks, CA: Sage Publications Inc: 3–34.

Popova, M. (2016) *Diane Ackerman on the Evolutionary and Existential Purpose of Deep Play*. Online. HTTP: <www.brainpickings.org/2016/08/04/diane-ackerman-deep-play/> (accessed 20 November 2019).

Public Library of Science (2016) *Similarities Found in Bee and Mammal Social Organization*. Online. HTTP: <https://phys.org/news/2016-06-similarities-bee-mammal-social.html> (accessed 5 November 2019).

Radford, T. (2019, 31 October) The rise of the greedy-brained ape. *Nature*, 574: 623–625.

Rosen, S. (2010) *My Voice Will Go with You: The Teaching Tales of Milton H. Erickson*. New York: W.W. Norton.

Royal Shakespeare Company (2019) *As You Like It: Synopsis*. Online. HTTP: <www.rsc.org.uk/as-you-like-it/the-plot> (accessed 27 November 2019).

Schwertly, S. (2014) *The Neuroscience of Storytelling*. Online. HTTP: <www.cavill.com.au/wp-content/uploads/2016/08/Ethos-3-2014-The-Neuroscience-of-Storytelling.pdf> (accessed 5 July 2019).

Sloan, M. M. (2018) What made ancient Greeks special? Storytelling. *Wakeforest Magazine*. Online. HTTP: <https://magazine.wfu.edu/2018/03/28/lessons-from-the-greeks-and-romans-2/> (accessed 18 June 2019).

Storlie, J. (2014) *Difference between a Case Study and a Story?* Online. HTTP: <www.linkedin.com/pulse/20141022015045-35908278-difference-between-a-case-study-and-a-story> (accessed 20 November 2019).

Storr, W. (2019) *The Science of Storytelling*. New York: William Collins.

Storytelling Brands (2019) *Telling Stories: Communicating in Symbols and Pictures*. Online. HTTP: <www.newbrandstories.com/2011/05/26/telling-stories-communicating-in-symbols-and-pictures/> (accessed 15 November 2019).

Tonkin, A. and Whitaker, J. (Eds.) (2016) *Play in Healthcare for Adults: Using Play to Promote Health and Wellbeing across the Adult Lifespan.* Oxon: Routledge.

Walters, R. (2017) Fairytales, psychodrama and action methods: Ways of helping traumatized children to heal. *Zeitschrift für Psychodrama und Soziometrie*, 16 (1): 53–60.

Westenberg, J. (2017) *Storytelling Is the Number One Skill You Have to Improve.* Online. HTTP: <https://inc42.com/entrepreneurship/storytelling-skill-improve/> (accessed 29 November 2019).

Winterson, J. (2011) *Why Be Happy When You Could Be Normal?* London: Vintage.

Zeig, J. (1980) *A Teaching Seminar with Milton H. Erickson.* New York: Brunner/Mazel.

3 Infancy and the early years

The first 1000 days of human life, from conception to two years of age, have been described as 'a unique period of opportunity when the foundations of optimum health, growth, and neurodevelopment across the lifespan are established' (Cusick and Georgieff n.d.). By the end of this period, which has been identified as a key developmental assessment point, growth markers are predictive of subsequent intelligence and school performance in high-, middle-, and low-economic settings (Villar et al. 2019). As the foundation for learning (Piazza et al. 2020), play during the first 1000 days 'is not frivolous: it is brain building' (Yogman et al. 2018). Play at the start of life is not a trivial or frivolous matter because not only is it one of the building blocks for lifelong learning, but it is also a crucial factor in how well – and perhaps even how long – a person will live (Nijhof et al. 2018).

The first thousand days

At birth, the human brain is hardwired with all the neurons it will need throughout life, although the newborn infant is relatively immature when compared to other species since significant brain development continues after birth (Yogman et al. 2018). By the end of a child's first year, the brain will have doubled in size and by two years of age the brain has twice as many synapses as an adult brain (Urban Child Institute 2020). This rapid rate of brain growth, together with high levels of brain plasticity (Cusick and Georgieff n.d.), results in the fastest rates of physical, cognitive, and emotional development of any time during the life course. Play is fundamental to this developmental process because it is through play that the child explores their world and learns to communicate with confidence and to relate to those around them (Foundation Years 2019).

A recent study by Villar et al. (2019) has demonstrated that, at two years of age, neurodevelopmental milestones and their associated behaviors are similar across different cultures and diverse geographical regions. This matches the pattern of skeletal growth in healthy infants who are born to healthy mothers and who are well nourished throughout the first 1000 days. The developmental outcomes linked to these neurodevelopmental milestones include gross and fine motor skills, cognitive ability, receptive and expressive language, positive and negative behaviors, and emotional reactivity (Villar et al. 2019). The development of the cerebral cortex supports cognitive functionality, while it is the limbic system located deep within the inner brain which is related to the more instinctive behaviors such as emotional reaction and the reward-seeking behaviors associated with play (Urban Child Institute 2020). Panksepp (cited in Yogman et al. 2018) suggests that 'play is 1 of 7 innate emotional systems in the midbrain' and produces a young mammalian brain that is instinctively motivated to engage in playful behavior (Siviy 2016).

Play follows its own developmental trajectory, beginning with social smiling around the age of six weeks and progressing to reciprocal 'serve-and-return' interactions in which parents mimic baby's 'oohs and aahs' in back-and-forth verbal games. This leads to early conversational exchanges in which the infant participates in reciprocal vocalization, nurturing the development of early language skills (Yogman et al. 2018). By nine months of age, repetitive games such as Peek-a-boo and 'Round and Round the Garden' (Opie and Opie 1969) enable children to predict what is about to happen, indicating the emergence of self-regulation and impulse control, as well as the ability to elicit social stimulation from others.

By 12 months of age, the emergence of locomotor skills prompts rough-and-tumble play, allowing infants to experiment with risk in a safe and rewarding manner, nurturing negotiation skills and the development of emotional balance (Yogman et al. 2018). Research undertaken by Piazza et al. (2020) has demonstrated the neural coupling that occurs at this stage, whereby the brain and behavior of the infant shape and reflect that of their adult playmate through social cues such as gazing and smiling. This alignment between infant and adult brains demonstrates the important role of trusted caregivers who can act as a safe reference point during early exploratory play (Yogman et al. 2018).

In recent years, the integration of neuroscientific knowledge and psychosocial awareness has further enriched our understanding of how children develop during their first 1000 days. Piaget's concept of a first *sensorimotor* stage of development still dominates Early Years provision for infants, supporting the contemporary emphasis on physical activity as crucial for healthy brain development (Cambridge Childhood Partnership 2017). The World Health Organization (2019) has identified optimal levels of physical activity, sedentary behavior, and sleep for all healthy children under five years of age. Promoting the value of floor-based play and a 'the more the better' approach (World Health Organization 2019), it recommends that infants under a year old should spend at least 30 minutes per day engaged in physical play. This needs to include play in the prone position ('tummy time') which facilitates the strengthening of head, neck, shoulder, and trunk muscles and paves the way to physical activity milestones such as rolling over (at 4 to 6 months), crawling (from 5 to 11 months), and taking those first important steps around the age of 12 months (Gooey Brains 2015). Tummy time also offers an ideal opportunity for the 'playful interactions that encourage young children to respond to, or mimic adults' (Department for Education 2020).

Children aged between one and two years need to experience a variety of differing physical play activities, for a recommended minimum of 180 minutes per day (World Health Organization 2019). With increased mobility and independent movement, purposeful play becomes more naturally active, contributing to the child's cognitive, social, and emotional health and wellbeing (Gooey Brains 2015). During the child's second year, they might begin to play alongside others, venturing further afield within a safe and emotionally secure environment (Department for Education 2020). At this stage it is important that play activities 'invite rather than compel participation' (Ministry of Education 1996: 40) so that children are free to develop at their own pace and according to their own interests and motivations.

The early years of childhood

Piaget's second stage of cognitive development is the *pre-operational* stage, which occurs between two and seven years of age, although its duration is contested as Piaget's methodology often led to an underestimation of children's cognitive capabilities (Smith 2010). During this stage, children learn to form internal representations; they are able to verbalize their thoughts, and thinking is intuitive as opposed to logical (Aspiranti 2011). Piaget (1976: 11) acknowledged that his *stage theory* is 'impossible to understand if one does not begin by analyzing in detail the biologic presuppositions from which it stems and the epistemological [knowledge] consequences in which it ends'.

The observations which led Piaget to view development as a series of distinct stages have subsequently been validated by increasingly sophisticated imaging techniques which show how development during the early years of childhood continues to be characterized by 'dynamic and elaborative anatomical and physiological changes' (Brown and Jernigan 2012: 313). Functional changes (such as symbolic representation, including symbolic play) reflect simultaneous regional and hemisphere-specific changes in the brain. An increase in the size of the cortex (which is associated with higher-order functions like language and information processing) is linked to alterations in interregional connectivity which are manifest in the inquiring, exploratory behavior typical of young children, who begin to use questions and experimentation to solve problems. At this stage, a greater number of brain regions are involved in the completion of cognitive tasks, in comparison to later stages of development. This suggests that 'scaffolding' (a framework to support adaptability) facilitates the organization of early cerebral functioning, with the scaffolding being dismantled as the child gets older (Brown and Jernigan 2012).

Physiologically, this developmental epoch is characterized by the extension of fine and gross motor skills which leads to increased independence and enhanced physical capability, enabling children to play and explore more freely of their own volition. *Playing and Exploring* is one of three 'effective characteristics of learning' in the Early Years Foundation Stage in England, which emphasizes the importance of play for healthy, holistic development (Department for

Education 2020). *Realising the Ambition* (Education Scotland 2020a), Scotland's revised practice guidance for the early years, acknowledges that play and relationships are central to a child-centered pedagogy, which offers all children an equal chance to achieve their developmental potential. And in Wales, the Foundation Phase developmental curriculum, which applies to all children between three and seven years of age, is based on the principles of learning through play and ties in with the Welsh government's commitment to creating a *Play Friendly Country* (gov.wales 2014), which recognizes the importance of play 'in laying the foundation for each child in reaching their full potential during their adult life' (Gething cited in gov.wales 2014).

The song and dance of attachment and separation

Healthy development from the very start of life depends on two related psychological processes – attachment and separation – which we now examine in more detail. Both of these processes are supported by the play relationship and represent the first steps on a timeline of connection.

Parent and child face two crucial tasks during the first stage of their life together. The first of these is to form a close attachment bond, within which the child can grow the trust necessary for all future relationships. The second is to use this attachment as a secure base from which to learn to separate from one another in order for the child to be able to develop a sense of selfhood (Marvin et al. 2002). Play has a role as a mediator in both these processes: it supports the development of secure attachment, and attachment supports the development of play. James (2016: 59) sums it up: 'Along with the gold dust of creativity and playfulness, it is out of satisfying our children's need for dependence that their independence is born'.

Attachment is primarily an evolutionary process which emerged as a result of natural selection: it is a simple matter of survival. Young mammals who stay close to an attachment figure are more likely to receive nourishment and protection and are therefore more likely to survive into adulthood. It has been described as 'the most pervasive mechanism in early childhood because it is a highly evolutionarily effective indicator of trustworthiness' (Fonagy and Luyten 2018). The related concept of *mentalization* has extended our understanding of attachment in human infants by emphasizing the significance of 'mind-to-mind' interaction in the parent–child relationship. The ability to recognize and interpret the meaning behind one's own feelings and behavior, as well as those of others, is key to self-differentiation and to the development of self-awareness (Bowen 1974) – and 'it depends not only on genes and the brain, but also on lived experiences, subjectivity, texts, discourse, and interpretations' (Karterud and Kongerslev 2019). It depends on early positive interaction.

Early play starts with a song: the sound of the mother's voice – which has been described as an auditory fingerprint that activates her child's brain, not just in infancy but throughout life (Fehlhaber 2020). The manner in which babies and mothers engage in vocal exchange is inherently playful: interactions are self-generated, motivated, and reinforced by curiosity and pleasurable feedback and include creative and diversional features (Ferguson 1964). Even before birth, the growing child responds to the mother's voice, and talking and singing to the baby is often the first of the bonding behaviors. Within hours of birth, the baby can differentiate the mother's voice and makes efforts to hear it better; the sound of her voice is reassuring to the newborn. It reduces stress by lowering cortisol levels and increases the production of oxytocin, the trust hormone, 'enhancing the mother–infant bond and promoting infants' social, emotional, and cognitive development' (Trehub 2017).

Shortly after birth, the infant starts to show interest in the mother's face as well as her voice and so begins 'the dance' of early play. Mutual eye gaze is central to communication and is a key feature of both maternal sensitivity and infant attachment security (Meltzoff and Brooks 2007). Babies have been shown to imitate facial gestures within hours of birth, and when the mother mirrors her baby's own facial expressions, she accepts an invitation to join the dance that is emotional synchrony. Parental engagement in 'the song and dance' of attachment play acknowledges the child as a separate being with intentions, motivations, and emotions distinct from their own, while the reciprocity of playful interaction affords the baby a sense of both understanding and of being understood – essential for the development of theory of mind, which is fundamental both for social interaction and for the formation of a strong sense of self.

Play originates deep within the human brain and deep within the human soul: it is a hallmark of our very humanity (Ackerman 1999). As an expression of love and connection, play both creates and sustains new life; a first step on the yellow brick road to personhood.

The child who misses out on playful interaction at the start of life is denied the opportunity to explore and validate their mental states, disrupting the development of a capacity for self-reflection and emotional regulation. Babies need 'responsive love' (James 2016: 105) which involves the parent or caregiver being fully present in an interaction if they are to 'tune in' to the infant's desire for connection. There is now emerging evidence that the pervasive use of smartphones by parents risks impacting negatively on opportunities for these crucial early deep play connections (Raudaskoski et al. 2017) with potentially devastating implications for child development. We have argued elsewhere (Whitaker 2019) that attachment play in early childhood is fundamental for the development of both empathy and self-compassion, two processes which are essential not only for individual health and wellbeing but for the creation of healthy communities.

The following case-stories illustrate two different approaches to supporting the attachment relationship through playful interaction. Challenging social circumstances demand novel and creative mediation, and play can be a gateway to new connections. In the first of the case-stories, Julia describes a simple therapeutic intervention with far-reaching benefits.

Box 3.1 Neonatal Storytime: it's never too early to play

Julia Whitaker

Walking onto a neonatal intensive care unit (NICU) has been described as 'like landing on another planet' (Bliss 2020): the sights, sounds, medical procedures, and space-age equipment can be overwhelming for the uninitiated. I had been employed as a hospital play specialist for just a few years when I was asked to explore the possibility of offering a therapeutic play service to the NICU of the hospital where I worked. Research showing that 'the development of secure attachment can be compromised when infants are born preterm' (Gerstein et al. 2015) advocates such a multi-professional model of family-centered care.

In contrast to the noisy activity of the children's ward, the ambiance of the NICU was unexpectedly muted; hushed conversations interrupted only by the eerie bleeping of alarms. The finger play, massage, and lullabies that typified my interactions with babies on the children's ward seemed inappropriate to this hallowed setting and, as I moved gingerly between the incubators, I puzzled over what I could possibly have to offer these tiny miracles of nature. The incubators' fragile occupants and their tired, anxious parents looked as though the last thing they needed was to play!

On the children's ward, I often read stories to patients of all ages – as a distraction during blood tests and transfusions; to pass the time during the wait for surgery; and as a way of establishing a relationship with a shy newcomer. Reading stories can often bridge the gap when conversation falters or a child is too weak or anxious to play. As I thought about the parents watching over their babies in the NICU for hours on end, distanced from them both physically and emotionally, I wondered whether storytelling might breach a gap in connection (Flacking et al. 2012).

I started to take picture books on my forays into the NICU and so began what became known as 'Neonatal Storytime'. At first, I would read to the babies – much less embarrassing than 'baby talk' or singing – but parents were soon inspired to follow my example. Starting with old favorites such as Sam McBratney's *'Guess How Much I Love You'* and Debbi Gliori's *'No Matter What'* and working through Roger Hargreaves' *Mr Men* books and Jill Murphy's tales of *The Large Family*, we gradually expanded our catalogue. Parents would suggest or bring new books to add to the collection and we soon had a small 'neonatal library' at the entrance to the unit. The familiar activity of reading or telling a story served to soften the sharp corners of a NICU stay and opened the door to play.

It was many years after my stint in the NICU that I came across research from Georgetown in the US (cited in Cox Gurdon 2019) which showed that not only does reading to babies in the neonatal period promote 'better interaction between parent and child' (Abubakar cited in

Cox Gurdon, 2019: 52) but that premature babies register fewer physiological fluctuations during and immediately after being read to by their parents (*ibid.*). Neonatal Storytime engages parents and their babies in an emotionally synchronous interaction which nourishes the attachment relationship, reducing stress, increasing closeness, and establishing playful connections from the very start of life.

The devolved administrations in the UK, along with combined authorities in England, have become increasingly aware of the impact of arts-based strategies to address the social determinants of health and wellbeing. The All Party Parliamentary Group on Arts Health and Wellbeing (2017) has explored how arts engagement can reduce the impact of health inequalities throughout the life course, and the following case-story describes one initiative which takes up the challenge of giving every child a fair chance of achieving 'the best start in life' (Marmot 2010).

Box 3.2 Expecting Something: a creative play and arts project for young families

Starcatchers

Starcatchers is Scotland's National Arts and Early Years Organization specializing in creating exceptional arts and creative experiences for babies, toddlers, and young children aged 0–5. As well as creating live theatre, dance and music performances, and arts installations, Starcatchers delivers engagement projects across Scotland, placing artists directly into the heart of communities.

Expecting Something has been active since 2014 in two localities which are characterized by social exclusion and high levels of poverty. During regular weekly sessions, the project offers opportunities for young parents (16–25 years) and their babies (0–2 years) to engage in creative play and arts activities together, which they would not otherwise have access to. Facilitated by professional artists, the aim of the project is to build parental confidence, strengthen parent–child bonds, and encourage supportive peer relationships.

The *Expecting Something* program is about expectations: the expectation that anyone can play and create, regardless of their life circumstances, and the expectation that anyone can connect, given the opportunity. Early in life, social connections make neural connections. The brain's architecture is partially shaped by early interactions with others and positive, responsive interactions between birth and three years of age can provide a strong foundation for connections that form later (Center on the Developing Child 2020).

Expecting Something takes parents on a creative journey with their little ones. As they grow in confidence week by week, parents discover a new-found playfulness in family life and continually make new discoveries about their babies' personalities, capabilities, and interests – while having fun in the process. 'Taking part in artistic and creative activities together is protected time for parents and their children, when they can really focus on being together, strengthening relationships and encouraging deeper bonds' (*Expecting Something Project Coordinator*).

Parental feedback reveals the insight that arises from playing together: 'I liked making the dreamcatchers. I liked it 'cause Gregor would go and get me a piece of material and he would wait until I'd cut the piece of material and put it on and then he would go find me another piece. So, it was really working together, he's still got it in his room now. That was really nice to be able to design that and do that together'.

Kyle was showing early signs of autism. He disliked being near other people and was overly sensitive to music, which could trigger a stress response. At one *Expecting Something* session, the group were visited by an African musician with a djembe drum and Kyle's mother watched awestruck as her son cautiously approached the musician while he beat out a rhythm on the drum. When the drumming stopped momentarily, Kyle picked up the musician's hands replacing them on the drum to indicate that he wanted more. As the rhythm resumed, Kyle did a little circle dance of appreciation, holding the attention of all those present. Play needs no words! After six months of participating in *Expecting Something* sessions, Kyle's mother was enabled to see him in a new light – as a whole person who could exercise choice and who held the power to make things happen.

Although parenthood is a positive experience for many young people, it is associated with increased risk of a range of poor social, economic, and health outcomes for some. Good-quality, integrated support for young parents and their families contributes to better engagement with support services and, in the longer term, greater engagement in education, training, and employment. This in turn will contribute to improved health and social outcomes for young parents and their children.

Playing 'with wonder'

The potency of play for creating the connection that supports the development of secure attachment and separation in the early years may be explained in part by the associated sense of awe and wonder it elicits in both the child and the parent (L'Ecuyer 2019). In the aforementioned case-story, Kyle's mother is described as 'awestruck' as she observes her usually detached son engage *with wonder* in a musical interaction. Parents everywhere will be able to identify examples of this 'wondering' in their own infants; when they discover their own fingers and toes, as they reach for a sunbeam, as they create a splash in a puddle. Awe and wonder are vital for healthy development because they inspire curiosity (Bersanelli and Gargantini 2009), and it is this curiosity which stimulates the pleasure center of the brain, the *nucleus accumbens*, flooding the brain with feel-good hormones and boosting physiological and emotional regulation systems. Recent studies (e.g., Keltner 2016; Rudd et al. 2012) have identified compelling correlations between the experience of awe and improved health, a sense of location in time and place, and an increase in pro-social behaviors such as kindness, cooperation, and resource-sharing – as well as enhanced critical and creative thinking faculties.

L'Ecuyer (2019: 13) writes that awe and wonder '[allow] us to transcend our everyday existence in order to experience it', echoing Huizinga's (1998) conceptualization of play as something *out of the ordinary*, detached from everyday life yet integral to it. In the next case-story, Jenni Etchells communicates the sense of 'magic' and wonder which she discovered through involvement in another arts-based initiative, *Hartbeeps©*. Sharing this experience with her baby helped Jenni to bond with her daughter, while also offering moments of respite from the overwhelming demands of new parenthood.

Box 3.3 Hartbeeps©: taking a magical journey into the imagination

Jenni Etchells

When inside the bubble of new parenthood, there is so much to think about. Advice seems to come from all directions and, however well-intended, it can often feel untimely and overwhelming. One of the highlights of the first year of Grace's life, and a welcome respite from everyday concerns, was the weekly *Hartbeeps©* class we signed up to when she was eight weeks old. This program offers 'innovative, multi-sensory and highly interactive productions for the very young' deploying music, sound effects, songs and sound plays, lighting effects, props, and puppetry to transform everyday environments into an imaginary world (Hartbeeps© 2020).

The *Hartbeeps©* sessions represented 45 minutes each week when we could hide away in a side room at the local soft play center to be transported to a magical land where all inhibitions faded away as I bonded with Grace through music, touch, and play. I would lay her down on the makeshift green 'grass', remove my shoes, and sit down beside her; Grace would turn her head to stare at the babies on either side of her, sometimes smiling, sometimes reaching out to them, and occasionally blowing a raspberry! At around three to four months of age, Grace began to roll over to assess each of her little 'classmates' before the music started. This gave me a chance to greet a neighboring parent, or a grandparent who had been brought along on our make-believe journey, whether that was to the seaside, to the park, or to the shops. The teacher would gently guide the class into the land of *Hartbeeps©*, repeating the same songs from week to week and using carefully chosen props linked to a weekly theme. Finger-puppets were a firm favorite, alongside egg shakers and scarfs, which we used to play 'peekaboo' or to waft over our baby's face as they explored color and texture through play.

When Grace moved to the class for older babies at six months of age, the props and songs changed, along with the ability of the babies to move around the room. As a parent, you might find yourself singing to someone else's child who had opted to sit on your lap. At the outset, this class seemed messy, loud, and chaotic: some babies fed throughout the session, some cried, and some chose to have a nap on the grass. However, this meant you learned to accept and respond to your child's needs and felt encouraged to bring your baby to the sessions, regardless of whether they were teething, having a growth spurt, or just having a grumpy day. There was never any judgment and no pressure for the babies to take part in the structured aspects of the class if they chose not to. Each week, the teacher reminded parents that babies are still taking everything in, even when they are feeding and sleeping – a valuable lesson to take back to everyday life.

Some weeks, Grace would play happily for the duration of the class, giggling with glee as we pretended to be on a farm. At other times, she would sit quietly on my lap, watching the other children play, just taking in what was going on around her. Every week I would take home new ideas for how to interact with Grace and we steadily built up a repertoire of different ways to play and bond together. Grace is now four years old, but the magic of *Hartbeeps©* has stayed with us: the songs which we learned in class, together with elements of baby massage and other calming techniques, became part of our bedtime routine and have been revived since her baby sister came along. We recently returned to *Hartbeeps©* as a threesome – a noisier and more energetic experience in the preschool class, but equally magical. It is humbling to allow your child to take you to their world through play and to be reminded to set your inhibitions aside to enter and interact with them in their world.

The gift of nature

L'Ecuyer (2019: 52) states that 'nature is one of the first sparks to light the flame of wonder in a child' and play in nature is perhaps the greatest gift that adults can give to a young child. In his bestselling book, *Last Child in the Woods*, Richard Louv (2009) presents the powerful case that direct exposure to nature is essential for healthy childhood development and for the physical and emotional health of both children and adults. Play in nature offers opportunities for the all-important physical play outlined at the start of this chapter and stimulates the natural curiosity by which children learn about themselves and the world around them. Perhaps most importantly, play feeds the sense of wonder that connects the child to the earth, such that they become part of something greater even than themselves and can face the future in the certain knowledge, 'that with each of them all things are remade, and the universe is put again upon its trial' (Chesterton cited in L'Ecuyer 2019: 11). The next case-story by Elizabeth Henderson exemplifies perfectly the young child's oneness with the natural world.

Box 3.4 From nature comes nurture: growing empathy and resilience

Elizabeth Henderson

Snails appeared frequently in the nursery garden and woodland – a consequence of our wet climate combined with a number of rocks and stones that afforded them shelter. Children often recoiled on seeing the snail's feelers disappear and grimaced at the snail's stickiness. However, they gazed in amazement too when the snail's feelers popped out of the shell again and the snail moved on, leaving its silvery trail behind.

'How does it do that?' they would ask, watching in wonder. Jacob, however, on seeing snails for the first time simply stamped on them and laughed as he broke their shells, squishing them into the ground and oblivion.

I quietly gasped at his forcefulness and his lack of care and curiosity about the snails, except that is to see if he could overpower them. My first thought was 'Why?' yet I already knew the answer to that.

Jacob seemed to lack empathy and was, instead, quite ruthless with living things, leaving a trail behind him of broken flower-heads, stone-beaten snails, and battered berries. Knowing the challenges in his life, however, I understood why he might feel a need to control and hurt others, for that was what he had experienced at home.

Theories of neural development informed me that Jacob's mirror neurons would emulate what he had seen and the subsequent process of embodiment, over a period of time, would shape his identity and behaviors, negatively. However, I firmly believed that nature could impact on this process too – but I was having a problem getting this over to my colleagues and other children's parents, who frequently raised their concerns with me about Jacob's destructiveness.

As an environment, nature provides a nonthreatening and nonaggressive context in which children can absorb new experiences: nourish their senses; feel a freedom in their bodies; take risks climbing, jumping, rolling, falling; find refuge in a secret den; wonder at ever-evolving and changing colors in the landscape; and develop a sense of ownership and belonging by naming a space, making it *their* place – 'the pirate tree' or 'blackberry land'. By late wintertime, however, I was struggling with the stress of Jacob's needs when suddenly the snow began to fall, muffling sounds and dusting everything with white magic.

Later that day we played in the woods, for what seemed like forever, making snow animals. Uncharacteristically Jacob quietly gathered snow, moving back and forth from his chosen snow heap, alone. Then, suddenly, he seemed to take a long time to return, so I went over to investigate.

Brushing snow gently aside, he had revealed tiny green shoots, some with tight buds. Hearing my footsteps, he pointed and shouted, 'What's that?'

'They're snowdrops' I replied, 'and when they open, they look like snow-bells'.

He gasped and turned his face toward me, his eyes wide open in amazement.

'Snowdrops, snow-bells?' he repeated. He crouched down and gently stroked them before asking, 'Who put them there?'

Snowdrops – nature's gift to Jacob.

Movement is the basis for all development, and physical play at the start of life nurtures and promotes the complex interplay of brain, body, and mind (Schweizer 2009). Young children are naturally drawn to interact physically with their environment, developing an understanding of the world and their connection to it through the senses. From an early age, they need the time, space, and adult encouragement to explore and experiment using their whole body. Moving in relation to the earth – crawling, balancing, climbing – fosters spatial awareness. Walking, running, and jumping develop muscle strength and coordination and build healthy lungs. Fine motor skills are refined through picking up and manipulating objects of different sizes and shapes. Physical play in the natural environment boosts the immune system, encourages a healthy appetite, and prepares the body for rest and sleep. It also allows children to learn to assess and manage risk, the experience of which is regarded as 'a foundation for life and [for] understanding themselves and their capabilities' (Little et al. 2012).

The concept of the Forest Kindergarten originated in Scandinavia in the 1950s and a growing awareness of the importance of outdoor play, and of the consequences of 'nature deficit disorder' (Louv 2009), has spurred the growth of outdoor early education provision throughout the UK (e.g., Education Scotland 2020b). Play in nature gives children the opportunity to grow and to learn in an ever-changing environment, offering them the best preparation for dealing with life in a fast-changing world, without losing their sense of wonder and connection. The following case-story offers a snapshot of play in a natural environment highlighting the various benefits for health and learning which have been discussed throughout this chapter.

Box 3.5 'I have never tried that before, so I think I should definitely be able to do that'

(Lindgren 2004)
Hilary Long

Climbing trees is a favorite activity for many of our children. Most of our camps have at least one good climbing tree. This is a four-year-old girl's first experience of climbing a tree.

This little girl beams with self-confidence. She masters the problem-solving process of foot and hand placement. She invites her friend to join her. Once up they proceed to play a game in the tree. They encourage and support one another. Together they enjoy the tactile experience of touching bark and leaves. Making enough room for one another involves spatial awareness. Using their innate wisdom, they descend safely. Children demonstrate the physical and intellectual skills required for tree climbing and enjoy the peaceful solitude that the perspective of a tree perch provides (Figure 3.1).

Rope swings are popular with the children. Making one involves much collaboration. Children choose the tree for branch strength and height. They like the log seat to be far enough off the ground so that their feet are clear of the woodland floor. Today the request is for some thrills and spills. Instead of the usual back and forward the request came from a three-year-old to go 'round and round very fast'. 'You'll get dizzy', I say. Staff demonstrate how to hold the rope tightly and set him off into the air. Round and round at increasing speed. Shrieking with delight, eyes tightly shut he finally shouts, 'stop my tummy is dizzy'.

Camps have large, upturned tree roots large enough for climbing but more often used for imaginative play. One has roots that have left a deep pit. Today a four-year-old boy is desperate to have a go at climbing up this. Different techniques are required as there are no proper branches to hang on to. We watch as he thoughtfully and carefully climbs to the top. A rope is suspended from a branch at the top for him to use to descend. Coming down the rope he loses his grip and falls into the pit. Slowly I walk toward him. "Are you ok" I say. He looks up at me and roars with laughter. "Can I do that again?" he says.

Children built a bridge across a stream. Some children prefer to cross by foot. A four-year-old girl gets stuck as the mud sucks her wellington boots down. Great excitement abounds as the rest of the group devise a plan to rescue her. With a member of staff at each end of the 'crocodile' together they pull her out. What delight when they see that she has left her boots behind. One child who had gathered stones to throw in the water looks up and sees the boots. "Where has O . . . gone?" he says. Laughter sounds throughout the woods.

"I love my outdoor nursery. It's very fun. I can't really remember everything about what I done but it feels just fun and lovely and nice playing with my friends . . . My cheeks are pink with oxygen!"

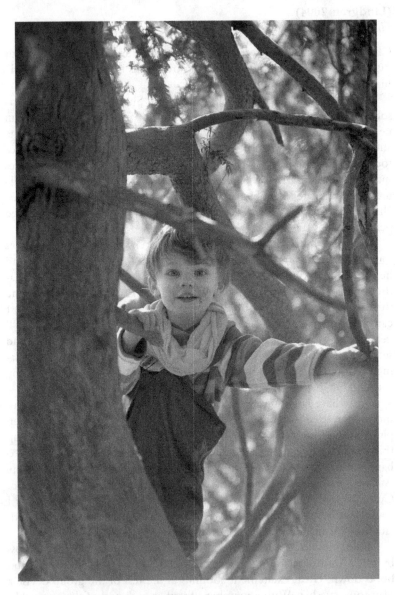

Figure 3.1 Climbing trees is a favorite activity

Source: Photograph by Hilary Long.

In *Realising the Ambition*, the national practice guidance for early years in Scotland, *Section 4: Child's work: the importance of play*, opens with the following quote from Froebel, widely acknowledged as the founder of the modern kindergarten movement: 'play at this time is not trivial, it is highly serious and of deep significance' (Education Scotland 2020a: 43). The guidance acknowledges that play is the medium through which the child learns best and that enabling a play pedagogy is a skillful job. The adult's role in the early years is to create an environment – physical, social, and emotional – that allows play and learning to happen alongside each other by inviting curiosity, offering new opportunities, and nurturing healthy growth.

In our final case-story for this chapter, experienced practitioner Alison Hawkins, who is the principal of Wester Coates Nursery School in Edinburgh, offers an insight into play pedagogy in practice.

Box 3.6 Roots and shoots: learning to 'live the day'

Alison Hawkins

'Come play today the Froebel Way!', sounds like a trite invitation to a magical session, suggestive of some fun and leisure as a one-off experience. It is, however, worth unpicking the meaning behind the phrase as it goes considerably deeper than it might appear.

Friedrich Froebel was born nearly 250 years ago, and it is his legacy upon which much of twenty-first-century Early Years Practice is based (Tovey 2017). Credited as the founder of kindergarten, Froebel saw children as unique, curious, motivated, and competent. Through his many detailed observations of children's lives, behaviors, and attitudes – spanning decades – he concluded that the learning of young children should be driven by them, with their interests at the fore and unrestricted by adult interference. Instead, he regarded adult contributions to be important in the context of supporting and extending experiences, but not as teacher-enforcers. He witnessed the deep engagement a child develops in their play and realized that is where understanding, problem-solving, and learning occurs best for young children. While each individual was valued, importance too was placed on community, and the rhythm of the days and the seasons of the year were fundamental in his thinking. Children learned to bake, to clean, to sew, and to craft objects with clay and wood. These skills empowered children to be self-sufficient. Being outdoors was regarded as natural and emphasized his thought that children need to be 'at one' with themselves and their world. Gardening was a prominent occupation and he considered that this 'work' led children to be confident in looking after themselves.

His 'garden for children' and his 'garden of children' are nowadays an oft-used analogy, as roots grow shoots and spread. Across the globe in the 2020s practitioners are researching, and subsequently embracing, the principles of play based on Froebel's approach and translated through the work of current theorists such as Tina Bruce (2015).

Wester Coates Nursery School (WCNS) is founded on such principles and the ethos echoes those early Froebelian teachings.

Our play is largely self-led, almost always outdoors, and is scaffolded by experienced staff. Children pursue their own play, or engage in group play, as is their want. Their play encompasses role play, physical play, experimenting with water, and building with blocks and open-ended materials; mark-making takes many forms – chalking, using a stick in mud, painting, and drawing. The beauty of their environment is acknowledged by watching the buds of spring and summer bloom, and fade in autumn and winter, and by observing the birds and wildlife around them. Being outdoors produces a calm in our children – and at times gives space to let off steam!

In keeping with the sense of strong community we gather a couple of times a day to exchange news, to sing, and hear or tell stories. Through this, children exercise recall and may process emotions – happy or sad. Our parent body and those with strong associations to the nursery endorse our practice and there exists a network of interested adults ready to give support when required.

We see WCNS as a large family, and as we play and learn we simply regard ourselves as 'living the day'.

Conclusion

Many challenges in adult society have their roots in the early years of life, including major public health concerns such as obesity, heart disease, and mental health problems (WHO Commission on Social Determinants of Health 2008). The critical importance of the first 1000 days for lifelong health, wellbeing, and life chances cannot be overstated (Marmot 2010), for it is during this period that the rapidly growing brain is most adaptive to its social and physical environment, making it 'both versatile and vulnerable' (Centre for Community Child Health 2017: 5). This is not to downplay the importance of subsequent life stages, for the process of human development is an organic one: 'the window of opportunity for its development does not close on a child's third birthday' but continues well into adolescence – and beyond (Harvard Center on the Developing Child 2016.)

Play is one of the most important ways in which infants and young children learn to adapt to their physical, social, and emotional environment and to acquire the knowledge and skills which will set them on course for a healthy life. From the golden template of early attachment and separation to creating opportunities for active exploration (especially in nature), play is considered to be a critical component in the development of cognitive, social, and emotional wellbeing, as well as physical development (Gooey Brains 2015). Establishing a 'habit of play' (Fahey 2015) from the very start of life opens the door to a lifetime of possibility.

References

Ackerman, D. (1999) *Deep Play*. New York: Vintage.

All Party Parliamentary Group on Arts Health and Wellbeing (2017) *Creative Health: The Arts for Health and Wellbeing: The Short Report*. London: All Party Parliamentary Group on Arts Health and Wellbeing.

Aspiranti, K. B. (2011) Preoperational stage (Piaget). In: Goldstein, S. and Naglieri, J. A. (Eds.), *Encyclopedia of Child Behavior and Development*. Boston, MA: Springer: 114.

Bersanelli, M. and Gargantini, M. (2009) *From Galileo to Gell-Mann: The Wonder That Inspired the Greatest Scientists of All Time*. West Conshohocken, PA: Templeton Foundation Press.

Bliss (2020) *Information for Parents: When You First Arrive on the Neonatal Unit*. Online. HTTP: <www.bliss.org.uk/parents/in-hospital/about-neonatal-care/when-you-first-arrive-in-the-unit> (accessed 3 February 2020).

Bowen, M. (1974) *Toward the Differentiation of Self in One's Family of Origin*. New York: Jason Aronson.

Brown, T. T. and Jernigan, T. L. (2012) Brain development during the preschool years. *Neuropsychology Review*, 22 (4): 313–333. https://doi.org/10.1007/s11065-012-9214-1.

Bruce, T. (2015) *Early Childhood Education*. London: Hodder Education.

Cambridge Childhood Partnership (2017) *Benefits of Physical Activity on the Whole Child*. Online. HTTP: <www.panco.org.uk/wp-content/uploads/2018/01/Physical-Infographic-Nov-17.pdf> (accessed 26 February 2020).

Center on the Developing Child (2020) *Brain Architecture*. Online. HTTP: <https://developingchild.harvard.edu/science/key-concepts/brain-architecture/> (accessed 25 April 2020).

Centre for Community Child Health (2017) *The First Thousand Days: An Evidence Paper*. Victoria, Australia: Centre for Community Child Health.

Cox Gurdon, M. (2019) *The Enchanted Hour: The Miraculous Power of Reading Aloud in the Age of Distraction*. London: Piatkus.

Cusick, S. and Georgieff, M. (n.d.) *The First 1,000 Days of Life: The Brain's Window of Opportunity*. Online. HTTP: <www.unicef-irc.org/article/958-the-first-1000-days-of-life-the-brains-window-of-opportunity.html> (accessed 22 February 2020).

Department for Education (2020) *Development Matters: Non-Statutory Curriculum Guidance for the Early Years Foundation Stage*. London: Department for Education.

Education Scotland (2020a) *Realising the Ambition: Being Me: National Practice Guidance for Early Years in Scotland*. Online. HTTP: <https://education.gov.scot/media/3bjpr3wa/realisingtheambition.pdf> (accessed 13 September 2020).

Education Scotland (2020b) *Forest Kindergarten Approach: Learning Outdoors with Confidence*. Online. HTTP: <https://education.gov.scot/improvement/learning-resources/

forest-kindergarten-approach-learning-outdoors-with-confidence/> (accessed 26 April 2020).

Fahey, R. (2015) *The Habit of Play*. Online. HTTP: <https://usplaycoalition.org/the-habit-of-play> (accessed 3 July 2020).

Fehlhaber, K. (2020) *How a Mother's Voice Shapes Her Baby's Developing Brain*. Online. HTTP: <https://aeon.co/ideas/how-a-mother-s-voice-shapes-her-baby-s-developing-brain> (accessed 19 November 2020).

Ferguson, C. A. (1964) Baby talk in six languages. *American Anthropology*, 66: 103–114.

Flacking, R., Lehtonen, L., Thomson, G., Axelin, A., Ahlqvust, S., Hall Moran, V., Ewald, U. and Dykes, F. (2012) Closeness and separation in neonatal intensive care. *Acta Paediatrics*. 101 (10): 1032–1037. doi:10.1111/j.1651-2227.2012.02787.x.

Fonagy, P. and Luyten, P. (2018) Attachment, mentalization, and the self. In: Livesley, W. J. and Larstone, R. (Eds.), *Handbook of Personality Disorders*. New York, NY: Guilford Press: 123–140.

Foundation Years (2019) *Child Development and Early Learning*. Online. HTTP: <https://foundationyears.org.uk/2019/08/child-development-and-early-learning/> (accessed 18 February 2020).

Gerstein, E. D., Poehlmann-Tynan, J. and Clark, R. (2015) Mother-child interactions in the NICU: Relevance and implications for later parenting. *Journal of Pediatric Psychology*, 40 (1): 33–44.

Gooey Brains (2015) *Physical Development*. Online. HTTP: <http://gooeybrains.com/physical-development/> (accessed 26 February 2020).

gov.wales (2014) *Wales: A Play Friendly Country*. Online. HTTP: <https://gov.wales/sites/default/files/publications/2019-07/wales-a-play-friendly-country.pdf> (accessed 14 October 2020).

Hartbeeps (2020) *Home*. Online. HTTP: <www.hartbeeps.com/> (accessed 22 April 2020).

Harvard Centre on the Developing Child (2016) *From Best Practice to Breakthrough Impacts: A Science-Based Approach to Developing a Brighter Future for Children and Families*. Online. HTTP: <http://46y5eh11fhgw3ve3ytpwxt9r.wpengine.netdna-cdn.com/wp-content/uploads/2016/05/From_Best_Practices_to_Breakthrough_Impacts.pdf> (accessed 10 July 2020).

Huizinga, J. (1998) *Homo Ludens: A Study of Play-Element in Culture*. Oxon: Routledge.

James, O. (2016) *Not in Your Genes: The Real Reasons Why Children Are Like Their Parents*. London: Ebury Publishing.

Karterud, S. W. and Kongerslev, M. T. (2019) A temperament-attachment-mentalization-based (TAM) theory of personality and its disorders. *Frontiers in Psychology*, 10: 1–17.

Keltner, D. (2016) *Why Do We Feel Awe? Mindful: Taking Time for What Matters*. Online. HTTP: <www.mindful.org/why-do-we-feel-awe/> (accessed 29 May 2020).

L'Ecuyer, C. (2019) *The Wonder Approach*. London: Robinson.

Lindgren, A. (2004) *Pippi Longstocking*. London: Oxford University Press.

Little, H., Sandsetter, E. B. and Wyver, S. (2012) Early childhood teachers' beliefs about children's risky play in Australia and Norway. *Contemporary Issues in Early Childhood*, 13 (4): 300–316.

Louv, R. (2009) *Last Child in the Woods: Saving Our Children from Nature-Deficit Disorder*. London: Atlantic Books.

Marmot, M. (2010) *Fair Society, Healthy Lives: The Marmot Review: Strategic Review of Health Inequalities in England Post-2010*. London: University College London.

Marvin, R., Cooper, G., Hoffman, K. and Powell, B. (2002) The circle of security project: Attachment-based intervention with caregiver-pre-school child dyads. *Attachment & Human Development*, 4 (1): 107–124.

Meltzoff, A. N. and Brooks, R. (2007) Eyes wide shut: The importance of eyes in infant gaze following and understanding other minds. In: Flom, R., Lee, K. and Muir, D. (Eds.), *Gaze Following: Its Development and Significance*. Mahwah, NJ: Erlbaum: 217–241.

Ministry of Education (1996) *Te Whāriki. He Whāriki Mātauranga mōngā Mokopuna o Aotearoa: Early Childhood Curriculum*. Wellington: Learning Media.

Nijhof, S. L., Vinkers, C. H., [. . .] and Lesscher, H. (2018) Healthy play, better coping: The importance of play for the development of children in health and disease. *Neuroscience and Biobehavioral Reviews*, 95: 421–429.

Opie, I. and Opie, P. (1969) *Children's Games in Street and Playground*. Oxford, MA: Oxford University Press.

Piaget, J. (1976) Piaget's theory. In: Inhelder, B., Chipman, H. H. and Zwingmann, C. (Eds.), *Piaget and His School*. Springer Study ed. Berlin: Springer: 11–23.

Piazza, E., Hasenfratz, L., Hasson, U. and Lew-Williams, C. (2020) Infant and adult brains are coupled to the dynamics of natural communication. *Association of Psychological Science* 31 (1): 6–17.

Raudaskoski, S., Valkonen, S. and Mantere, E. (2017) The influence of parental smartphone use, eye contact and 'bystander ignorance' on child development. In: Lahikainen, A. R., Mälkiä, T. and Repo, K. (Eds.), *Media, Family Interaction and the Digitalization of Childhood*. Cheltenham, UK: Edward Elgar: 173–184.

Rudd, M., Vohs, K. D. and Aaker, J. (2012) Awe expands people's perception of time, alters decision making, and enhances well-being. *Psychological Science*, 23 (10): 1130–1136.

Schweizer, S. (2009) *Under the Sky: Playing, Working and Enjoying Adventures in the Open Air*. East Sussex: Sophia Books.

Siviy, S. (2016) A brain motivated to play: Insights into the neurobiology of playfulness. *Behaviour*, 153 (6–7): 819–844.

Smith, J. (2010) *Talk, Thinking and Philosophy in the Primary Classroom*. Exeter: Learning Matters Ltd.

Tovey, H. (2017) *Bringing the Froebel Approach to Your Early Years Practice*. Oxon: Routledge.

Trehub, S. E. (2017) The maternal voice as a special signal for infants. In: Filippa, M., Kuhn, P. and Westrup, B. (Eds.), *Early Vocal Contact and Preterm Infant Brain Development: Bridging the Gaps between Research and Practice*. New York: Springer International Publishing: 39–54.

Urban Child Institute (2020) *Baby's Brain Begins Now: Conception to Age 3*. Online. HTTP: <www.urbanchildinstitute.org/why-0-3/baby-and-brain> (accessed 22 February 2020).

Villar, J., Fernandes, M., [. . .] and Kennedy, S. (2019) Neurodevelopmental milestones and associated behaviours are similar among healthy children across diverse geographical locations. *Nature Communications*, 10: 511. https://doi.org/10.1038/s41467-018-07983-4.

Whitaker, J. (2019) Play, attachment and the empathy-equity connection. In: Tonkin, A. and Whitaker, J. (Eds.), *Play and Playfulness for Public Health and Wellbeing*. Oxon: Routledge: 79–91.

WHO Commission on Social Determinants of Health (2008) *Closing the Gap in a Generation: Health Equity through Action on the Social Determinants of Health: Final Report of the WHO Commission on Social Determinants of Health*. Geneva, Switzerland: World Health Organization.

World Health Organization (2019) *Guidelines on Physical Activity, Sedentary Behaviour and Sleep for Children under Five Years of Age.* Geneva, Switzerland: World Health Organization.
Yogman, M., Garner, A., Hutchinson, J., Hirsh-Pasek, K., Michnick Golinkoff, R., Committee on Psychosocial Aspects of Child and Family Health and AAP Council on Communications and Media (2018) The power of play: A pediatric role in enhancing development in young children. *Pediatrics*, 142 (3): e20182058.

4 The school years

Middle childhood, the period between 6 and 12 years of age, has traditionally been seen as a period of static consolidation, sandwiched between the dynamic transformations associated with early childhood and with adolescence (DelGiudice 2017). Previously underappreciated (DelGiudice 2017) and labelled the 'forgotten years' (Mah and Ford-Jones 2012), middle childhood is now emerging as an important developmental stage in its own right (Ministry of Children and Youth Services 2017). Characterized by cognitive, physical, social, and emotional advances (Mah and Ford-Jones 2012), middle childhood is a time when

> [C]hildren are exploring who they are and who they want to be, establishing basic skills and health habits, grappling with puberty, physical changes and gender roles, making friendships and forming attitudes about the world they live in, and taking first steps toward independence.
>
> (Ministry of Children and Youth Services 2017: 7)

'It is a time rich in potential that is just waiting to be cultivated' (Mah and Ford-Jones 2012: 81).

As in early childhood, development during this period is a holistic and fluid process that is interconnected and dependent on each developmental domain (Ministry of Children and Youth Services 2017). As they move through the first years of school, children become physically stronger and better coordinated; they are increasingly aware of their own thoughts and emotions – and those of other people (Mah and Ford-Jones 2012). Language acquisition continues at an impressive rate, enhancing the ability to communicate with others, although it remains hard for children of this age to put their ideas and feelings into words. Play along with other forms of symbolic representation such as art, music, and drama are now the main channels for self-expression and communication (Ministry of Children and Youth Services 2017). With increasing opportunities to socialize with their peers, without the need for adult intervention (Ludicology 2020), children gradually develop their social and communication skills, increasing their sociality through their natural inclination for play. Play experiences during middle childhood form the seedbed of resilience and adaptability, enhancing children's sense of personal wellbeing (*ibid.*) and readiness for the world.

Brain development in middle childhood

The middle years of childhood mark the next significant phase of brain development, which 'heralds a global shift in cognition, motivation and social behavior, with profound and wide-ranging implications for the development of personality, sex differences, and even psychopathology' (DelGiudice 2017: 95). By the age of six years, the brain has almost reached its maximum size and throughout middle childhood it continues to adapt rapidly, particularly in relation to social learning (DelGiudice 2017). This period marks the start of Piaget's third stage of *concrete operations*, when thought processes become more logical and children use their knowledge and experience of the physical world to organize information – an important prerequisite of strategic thinking and problem-solving (Börnert-Ringleb and Wilbert 2018).

During this stage, there are two growth spurts that occur in the brain, the first between six and eight years of age which leads to enhanced hand–eye coordination and improvements in fine motor skills (Boyd and Bee 2012). There is also progressive brain maturation in the regions associated with sensory functions such as vision, hearing, and touch (Ministry of Children and Youth Services 2017) and further development in areas of the brain linked to language processing. The second developmental spurt occurs between 10 and 12 years of age, when the frontal lobes of the cerebral cortex lead brain development, enabling improvements in memory and cognitive functioning associated with logic and planning (Boyd and Bee 2012).

Physical changes in the brain also occur during middle childhood with a thickening of the cerebral cortex (the outer layer of the brain often called the 'grey matter') and thinning of white matter in specific brain regions (Ministry of Children and Youth Services 2017). Myelination (developing sheaths around individual axons that improve the conductivity of nerves), leads to improved brain functioning and, between the ages of 6 and 12 years, the parts of the brain linked to sensory, motor, and intellectual functions are almost completely myelinated (Boyd and Bee 2012). This results in increases in information processing speeds: children can now think and do things much more quickly.

Gender-specific brain changes

Any discussion of brain development during middle childhood needs to consider gender-specific changes in the brain and whether these have implications for how children play and learn (McCarthy 2016). At a biological level, the brains of male and female children are largely the same in early childhood, with only 'subtle distinguishing elements' (Eliot cited in Take Care Staff 2018). However, Brizendine (2011, 2007) has identified a sustained divergence in the development of the male and female brain from the age of three, after which differentiation in the signaling pathways leads to changes in specific brain regions. This coincides with children being able to discriminate by gender when environmental influences reinforce societal attitudes linked to toy preferences and the provision of play opportunities (Eliot, cited in Take Care Staff 2018).

McCarthy (2016: 361) promotes an alternative, multifactorial approach to differentiation in the brain, alluding to 'enduring neuroanatomical and physiological changes that profoundly affect behavior'. At a cellular level, differentiation in the signaling pathways may lead to changes in specific brain regions but, according to McCarthy, this results in 'mosaicism of relative maleness, femaleness and sameness through the brain' (*ibid.*). Joel and Vikhanski (2019: 5) also contest the notion of a classically male or female brain and agree that 'these differences mix together in each individual brain to create a unique mosaic of features'.

Decades of research into children's play preferences have consistently identified differences in the play of boys and girls, which have been attributed to a complex combination of biological and developmental–environmental components (City, University of London 2017), However, a 2017 study (Todd et al. 2017) showed that play preferences develop differently in boys and girls as they move through childhood. While the time spent playing with male-type toys increases as boys get older, the same pattern is not apparent for girls – although this may simply be indicative of greater gender equality in Western societies where most of the studies were conducted (Todd cited in City, University of London 2017). Joel and Vikhanski (2019) make the point that, while the evidence for gendered play preferences is consistently reported, any evidence of 'sameness' is generally disregarded. However, there is overall agreement that the play opportunities offered to boys and girls should not be restrictive in the skills they afford, 'so that all children can learn from play and not miss out on the associated benefits for their development' (Todd cited in City, University of London 2017).

Acknowledging that the developmental process is genetically initiated but shaped by experience (Mah and Ford-Jones 2012), DelGiudice (2017: 99) identifies the transition to middle childhood as a 'developmental switch point' resembling a *sensitive period* which 'amplifies both environmental and genetic effects' on the child. This 'switch point' is coordinated by the awakening of the adrenal glands between six and eight years of age and the secretion of increased amounts of androgens which have a major impact on brain functioning. Adrenal androgens can be converted to estrogen or testosterone in the brain, resulting in the organization of brain development along differentiated sexual trajectories (DelGiudice 2017). Along with the awakening of the ovaries/testes, these developments signal the beginning of puberty. This sexual differentiation of brain pathways occurs many years before the appearance of secondary sexual characteristics, resulting in the decoupling of physical and behavioral development. This makes the middle childhood years a relatively risk-free time for social exploration, learning, and play; a time when children learn to tease, joke, gossip, and develop social rules that will last a lifetime (DelGiudice 2017).

Play and learning

DelGiudice (2017) classifies middle childhood as a phase of *juvenility* which is associated with the intense learning often achieved through play. This is true of all social mammals, most notably primates. However, in the UK, as in many Westernized nations, the role of play has become peripheral to children's education, as the emphasis switches away from child-led inquiry and playful exploration to adult-led learning (OpenLearn 2016). This is an educational approach with a foot in the past.

When Shakespeare (2006) wrote the 'Seven Ages' soliloquy in 1603, he portrayed childhood in the guise of a reluctant 'school-boy' because, in Elizabethan times, school was a reality known only to the male of the species – a gender bias that, shamefully, still exists in many parts of the world (Care 2020), despite education being a universal right endorsed in Article 28 of the United Nations Convention on the Rights of the Child (UNICEF 2020). The concept of universal, compulsory education garnered gradual support in Europe between the sixteenth and nineteenth centuries, much of the impetus being religiously motivated, whether with the explicit intention of instilling a knowledge of the scriptures, or with the more covert desire to contain childish exuberance within narrow moral parameters. Peter Gray (2008) observes that 'with the rise of schooling, people began to think of learning as children's work', and it remains the case that school often represents a demarcation between children's work and children's play.

Shakespeare's schoolboy would have started his schooling at around seven years of age – two or more years later than most children in the UK and the US nowadays. While 88 per cent of countries worldwide have a school starting age of six or seven, children in England now start formal schooling, and the learning of literacy and numeracy, at the age of four (Palmer 2016). There is growing support for the extension of a play-based curriculum into the first stages of primary education (e.g., Too Much Too Soon n.d; Upstart n.d.) which recognizes play, not just as the best route to learning in early childhood, but as a key determinant of health and wellbeing throughout the life course and across socio-economic differentials.

In our first case-story for this chapter, 13-year-old Erin reflects on the meaning of play from the perspective of a child who is on the cusp of adolescence and makes a persuasive case for a later school starting age and more time for play.

Box 4.1 A PLAYSUASIVE ESSAY: why we need to start school later and play for longer

Erin

Play can be many things, but for me it means freedom. Freedom to move however I want. Freedom to make whatever sound I like.

Freedom to choose how I use my time. Play is a human right (International Play Association [IPA] 2020) because it is part of what makes us human. But it feels like that right is taken away as soon as you set foot in school. School means being told to sit still, not fiddle, be quiet, do as you're told. Even in the nicest school, with the nicest teachers, it feels like you have to give up a piece of your freedom. Education is also a human right (*ibid.*), but why does it have to mean giving up the freedom to play? And why, in the UK, does it mean being taken to school at the age of four or five, when you are still clinging on to your parent's hand.

The answer to this question is to do with history (Palmer 2016). The reason children start school at age four or five in the UK is because of decisions made in the Victorian era. During the Industrial Revolution, employers wanted to get as much work out of people as they possibly could and by getting children into school as early as possible, they could have them ready to work by the time they were 12. In this way, employers could kill two birds with one stone because they could get the mothers back to work sooner and have the children ready to work in the mills or go down the mines when they were just 12. But we no longer live in Victorian times.

The UK and the US are among just a few countries in the world where children start school when they are five or under (Palmer 2016). In many other countries world-wide, including the Scandinavian countries, children don't start formal schooling until they are six or seven, with a nursery or kindergarten stage before that – and in a kindergarten (which means 'children's garden') little children have the freedom to play for longer.

Some people worry that children who start school later will be behind those who start school aged four or five (Cornelissen and Dustmann 2019). But this is not the case (Palmer 2016). Others just expect too much of their children or don't know any different because they started school at an early age themselves. Another argument is that an early school start gives an advantage to children from poorer backgrounds (Administration for Children & Families 2019). But why should play not be that advantage? There's now lots of evidence that children learn just as much through play as they can from school – perhaps even more (Palmer 2016). Play is: 'pretending, acting, singing, building, hiding, seeking, chasing, painting' (DK 2006), and these are all things that teach children the skills they will need for school and throughout their lives.

That leads to another question: why should play stop even when you start school? Whether you are big or small, you still have a human right to play and can still learn a lot from playing. But when tests and homework take over, time for play seems to completely vanish.

Play and the imagination

During the preschool and first years of school, the child's use of symbols in their play becomes increasingly sophisticated, and this is reflected in the structure and content of their drawings. Drawing can be seen as a transition between symbolic play and the emergence of the imagination (Krampen 2013). The imagination is organic: it grows and changes with increasing knowledge and experience of the world (PBS Education 2020). Imaginative teaching and learning nurtures the ability to envision the possible in all things (Egan and Judson 2015) and enriches the child's capacity for creative thinking, which then influences their ability to learn across the curriculum.

Grace (aged 4 years 6 months) has not yet acquired the cognitive skills to combine, separate, or transform ideas, but her drawing (Figure 4.1) contains all the elements of a story, offering an insight into how a child of this age processes and retains information for future use. In the days preceding the making of this drawing, Grace had been warned against retrieving her kite from a reservoir where there had been a recent drowning. Still in the preoperational stage, Grace generalizes this novel piece of information to apply it to a familiar activity – splashing in puddles. Box 4.2 is a transcript of a conversation between Grace (G) and her grandma (GM) about the picture she has drawn.

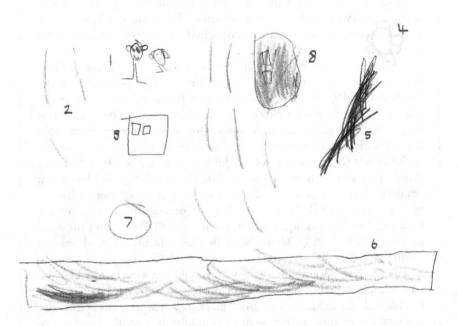

Figure 4.1 Creating early narratives

Source: Photograph by Alison Tonkin of an original drawing by Grace Etchells.

Box 4.2 Transcript of Grace's conversation with grandma

GM. *That's a lovely picture Grace. Can you tell me about it?*

G. *That's me and you (1) and we live there and it's really raining (2) and that's our house (3) and that's the sun (4).*

GM. *Fantastic – what's this? (5)*

G. *Nothing.*

GM. *And what about this? (6)*

G. *It's the swimming pool.*

GM. *The swimming pool – who goes in the swimming pool?*

G. *Me and You*

GM. *Me and You? Oh, that's lovely . . . and what's this here? (7)*

G. *Um . . . that's a puddle*

GM. *That's the puddle. . . . Do you jump in that with your wellies on?*

G. *No, because that's when you die.*

GM. *That's when you die? When you jump in the puddle? Oh dear! Does anyone else live in this house?*

G. *Daddy, Mummy and Emmy.*

GM. *Daddy, Mummy and Emmy. Fantastic . . . thank you. What's this Grace? (8)*

G. *That's our house.*

GM. *That's your house here . . .*

G. *That's the car . . .*

GM. *Whose car?*

G. *Yours.*

While drawing the picture, Grace was asked why Grandma's car had been colored pink, when it is actually black. Grace replied, *'I can decide to make it whatever color I like'* – and so she did!

Grace's story illustrates how storytelling can be a powerful tool for the reciprocal transmission of knowledge. One of the characteristics of middle childhood is the rapid and sustained development of episodic memory (DelGiudice 2017), which is reflected in the child's use of the imagination in their storytelling and in their play (Ministry of Children and Youth Services 2017). The next case-story demonstrates how trainee teacher, Victoria Webster, applied her knowledge of child development to playfully engage children during a classroom observation through the use of a simple artifact to ignite the children's imagination.

Box 4.3 Unlocking the imagination: using an artifact to inspire curiosity in a primary classroom

Victoria Webster

In my role as a trainee teacher, I was assigned the task of using an artifact to trigger curiosity and to facilitate interaction and discussion in a class of five- and six-year-olds. I decided to use the opportunity to employ a playful approach to inspire the children's imagination and to get them to 'think outside the box'. Encouraging children to use their imagination respects and values their own creative potential, freeing them to take risks and to state opinions rather than just search for correct answers.

My artifact was a key: a large, old-fashioned, golden key, quite different from the keys that the children might be familiar with. I concealed the key inside a bag and invited the children to feel it through the fabric of the bag, using the experience of 'not knowing' to engage their sensory curiosity. There was a palpable sense of anticipation as the bag was passed among the children waiting patiently for their turn to feel what might be inside. I invited them to think of a word/adjective to describe what they could feel and then to guess what it might be. The children were asked to keep their ideas to themselves until everyone had taken a turn, after which they were encouraged to share their speculations with the classmate sitting to the left of them and then with the whole class.

There was a gasp of astonishment when I opened the bag to reveal the key. I wondered aloud about the kind of door the key might open and asked the class: 'Using your imagination, what do you think this key would open and what would be behind the door?' As the children returned to their desks with paper and colored pencils to make a drawing of their ideas, there was a buzz of activity while they engaged enthusiastically with the task.

The drawings revealed magical gardens and treasure chests, but also some more elaborate fantasies. For one child, the key opened onto a secret passage which led to four secret galaxies, each depicted in detail. For another, the key opened a door into a magic world of sweets, with a lamp inhabited by a wish-granting genie. This child wished they could live in 'a massive house'. Another child's key unlocked a hairband containing a magical world. Yet another opened a window to reveal a rainbow world full of sparkly gems and unicorns. The atmosphere during the exercise was one of enjoyment and excitement as the children played around with their ideas.

Widespread recognition that play is 'the key' to children's learning (Palmer 2016) means that professionals in childhood care and education are obliged to develop the skills and knowledge necessary to become effective play advocates, including being able to articulate the value of play for lifelong health and wellbeing. Nicholson et al. (2013) have pointed out the irony that these play advocates typically have limited opportunities to incorporate play into their own lives. They suggest that it is only through creative, therapeutic, and meaningful play experiences in their adulthood that they will be able to 'develop the understanding and passion that will fuel their ability to courageously fight for children to have a right to play'. Stuart Brown (2008) warns that the alternative for 'those who play rarely' is that they 'become brittle in the face of stress or lose the healing capacity for humour'.

Playing through adversity

Learning to cope with challenge and adversity is an essential component of a healthy life (Lester and Russell 2014). Early research into 'resilience in the face of adversity' (Rutter 1985) identified the skills children need if they are to be able to manage stressful life experiences; these include the ability to assess and respond to risk and the flexibility to adapt to constantly changing circumstances – attributes which children develop through their play (Fearn and Howard 2012). The successful negotiation of life's ups and downs resides not in the evasion of risk but in successful engagement with it (*ibid.*), and play is perhaps one of the best modes of engagement.

Play is the child's natural medium of communication (Landreth 2002), and it is not mere serendipity that children often seek out play possibilities involving experimentation, jeopardy, and risk. Play which tests children to their physical and psychological limits activates a positive, biological stress response; we can say that, 'the ability and opportunity to play affords children a natural resource to meet [the] intellectual and emotional challenge[s]' which are part of grow-ing up (Fearn and Howard 2012: 456). When a child climbs to the uppermost branches of a tree, plays a game of 'Truth or Dare', or listens to a nail-biting ghost story, they are exercising this natural stress system (Dent 2003), and play which strengthens a child's natural coping mechanism encourages the healthy development of the whole child (Lester and Russell 2008). Sutton-Smith (2008: 119) concurs that children who have access to self-directed play and 'who enjoy ludic support for the whimsy of their inner lives are likely to be more sophisticated in their mature social lives and more diplomatically adept in their everyday social relations'.

In the following case-story, Kathrine Jebsen-Moore discusses how the changing face of play in the modern world denies many children this important aspect of their developmental agenda, with consequences for how they go on to navigate life's trials and tribulations.

Box 4.4 Free-range childhood: free play in an age of fear and control

Kathrine Jebsen-Moore

Oslo, 1985. Every morning, my mother would wrap me up in warm clothes and send me out the door, ready for my day at preschool. I would walk down our street, sometimes meeting old Anna on the cor-ner, out for a morning walk with her dog; she would stop and talk to me for a minute, before I walked on: past the big school, through the playing fields, across a small road, then up a small hill to the red-painted wooden building. It was about a kilometer in all, and we lived in a quiet and safe neighborhood in the suburbs of Oslo. I was five. Whenever I retell this story to fellow parents, they look at me in disbelief. This could never happen in Britain, they say. And I agree. Thirty-five years later, it would be unthinkable to send a five-year-old – or even a seven-year-old – outside the gate to venture unaccompanied to nursery or school.

Freedom became a prominent aspect of my childhood. And with no television until a half-hour at six o'clock, play was the order of the day. Either by myself, or with friends just a bike-ride or short walk away, or with my younger brothers. Outside or inside – there was no direction, but we were expected to behave sensibly. Common sense was developed as we grew and explored – mistakes were made, and looking back, there were occasions where I wonder if my parents were a bit naïve in their trust. But what happens when children are deprived of opportunities for free play, risk-taking, and self-direction?

Greg Lukianoff and Jonathan Haidt, authors of 'The Coddling of the American Mind' (2018), which explores how 'trigger warnings' and 'safe spaces' are doing more harm than good to today's university students, stress the importance of free play in a child's upbringing. Anxiety and other mental health issues among young people have risen sharply since the mid-nineties. Lukianoff and Haidt (*ibid.*) point to the rise of cable TV in the US in the 1980s, which exposed crimes such as kidnappings and made people scared of letting their children roam. Later, the internet and social media arrived. As a consequence, the generation born after 1994 (Generation Z) had more time indoors and less freedom, combined with more screen time, even as crime rates fell.

Children are anti-fragile, Lukianoff and Haidt (*ibid.*) say, and need to be exposed to some discomfort – like our immune systems – in order to develop properly. Although the real risk of serious danger has decreased, we have become used to thinking of children as vulnerable and potentially at risk. This, in turn, makes them more vulnerable, as we cocoon them to protect them. This vicious circle is hard to counteract.

Perhaps we tend to think back on our own childhoods with rose-tinted glasses, yet those experiences – playing in the stream, in the mountains, or cycling around my neighborhood – must be vivid memories for a reason. Perhaps part of the reason I remember them so fondly is that, although I was unaware at the time, these experiences helped me grow and mature. The need for children to play is still the same as it was a generation ago. We ought to be mindful of not just the importance of play, but of *free* play, and to remind ourselves that, although there are dangers out there, children are by nature hardy and resilient.

Resilience to challenge, change, and adversity can be understood as the outcome of an *interaction* between a child's personal attributes and the different features of their environment. 'During childhood, we are in constant dynamic interaction with our environment in a process of co-creation that drives physiological, cognitive and emotional development' (Fearn and Howard 2012). Play offers a safe passage through the tides of adversity because it provides opportunities for the development of the personal characteristics, skills, and capacities which are the building blocks of resilience (Pearson et al. 2017), while also contributing to the development of a 'protective environment' of positive relationships which can prevent or alleviate the damaging effects of toxic stress (Zhang et al. 2008).

Kenneth Ginsburg of The Children's Hospital of Philadelphia has identified what he has named the 'Seven Crucial Cs' of resilience: Competence, Confidence, Connection, Character, Contribution, Coping, and Control (Ginsburg and Jablow 2015). The *Play and Resilience* project of the World Organization for Early Childhood Development (OMEP) has accrued evidence from examples of best practice to identify the ways in which different forms of play interact to support Ginsburg and Jablow's 'Seven Cs' (2015) and consequently the development of physical and psychological aspects of resilience (Pearson et al. 2017) (see Table 4.1).

The challenges facing the twenty-first-century child may differ from those confronting previous generations, but they call on the same strengths, skills, and strategies that children have always needed as they move through the

Table 4.1 Play supports the development of personal and social resilience

Aspect of play	Personal resilience	Social resilience
Physical play (gross and fine motor)	Confidence and competence, through risk-taking and personal challenge. 'I can do this'.	Promotes cultural identity through social games, sports, music, and dancing.
Symbolic play (imitation, imagination)	Self-expression and the exploration of possibilities. 'I can be this'.	Promotes sense of identity and belonging through imitation of culturally specific roles and behaviors.
Object play (sensori-motor)	Problem-solving, decision-making, cooperation. 'We can work this out'.	Promotes a sense of belonging and cultural identification through the sharing of resources and responsibilities.
Socio-dramatic play	Negotiation, collaboration, conflict-resolution. 'We can overcome this'.	Allows for the experience of stress in a risk-free context and develops effective coping skills.
Games with rules	Sharing, turn-taking, Theory of Mind, persistence. 'This is who we are'.	Playing traditional/social games reinforces group identity and social cohesion.

Source: Adapted from Pearson et al. 2017.

world. Play is the bedrock on which healthy development is founded because it fosters each of the personal and social characteristics of resilience (Ginsburg and Jablow 2015).

The following case-story encompasses many of the elements identified in Table 4.1 and illustrates the way in which play contributes to Ginsburg and Jablow's 'Seven Cs'. Julia Findon describes one of the most eagerly awaited highlights of any camping trip by Cub Scouts – the campfire. Campfires have been described as the 'original social network' where people gather together to share stories through narratives, singing, drama, jokes, and games. At the end of the day, these 'fire-led activities centered on conversations that evoked the imagination, helped people remember and understand others in their external networks, healed rifts of the day and conveyed information about cultural institutions that generate regularity of behavior and corresponding trust' (Sugar Lake Lodge 2020).

Box 4.5 Creating memories: play around the campfire

Julia Findon

For Cubs and Scouts, camping provides an opportunity to engage with nature and to hone outdoor skills such as pitching and striking tents, building camp gadgets, while generally having fun. However, the highlight of any camp has always been the campfire, providing a chance for the whole camp to come together, be it a young person, a leader, or an adult helper.

The ritual of building the fire is an activity which will often take most of the day to prepare. To build an impressive fire which will last for several hours, mounds of firewood have to be carefully selected and collected, providing an opportunity for everybody to contribute to the evening's showpiece. Building the perfect campfire is quite an artform, and it often takes one or two seasoned experts considerable time to construct the focal point of the festivities, while at the same time passing on their knowledge to some young apprentices. The fire is usually constructed within a designated campfire circle, with seating in the form of benches and logs around the edges, although some campsites have a campfire circle that resembles a small amphitheater with the fire in the middle and stepped seating in a circle all the way round.

As dusk approaches, lit torches gradually appear through the gloom as people begin to gather around the fire and the noise levels rise excitedly as the time to light the fire approaches. Camp blankets are often worn, especially by the older members. These are blankets that are decorated with Beaver, Cub, and Scout badges that have been collected over time. As well as keeping the person warm, the badges are a reminder of many scouting moments and achievements over the years (Figure 4.2).

Once everyone has gathered, the fire is lit, and the campfire begins. A mixture of songs, skits (short comedy sketches which often parody the leaders), and stories play out against the backdrop of a roaring fire that lights up the night sky. The singing is usually led by one of the louder, more extrovert adults, with some quieter, more reflective, songs led by others. The songs cover many styles: some are thoughtful and sung softly, while others are more nonsense songs, and many have actions, which can get very silly. Then there are the 'yells', the most famous being 'Oggie Oggie Oggie' which requires the assembled gathering to yell back 'Oi, Oi Oi'. This is repeated several times . . . the louder the better.

A particular favorite at our campfires was the *Fried Chicken* song. The campfire leader would invite someone to join them and the pair would then engage in a shouting match, taking turns to yell as loud as they could 'I like fried chicken, I like fried chicken tonight'. As this was repeated over and over, the pair would skip around the campfire flapping their arms, before picking up another volunteer to join the yell. Before long, a chain of 'chickens' are skipping around the campfire, laughing, and flapping their wings, much to the amusement of the assembled gathering. Most people feel fine to make a fool of themselves – and usually

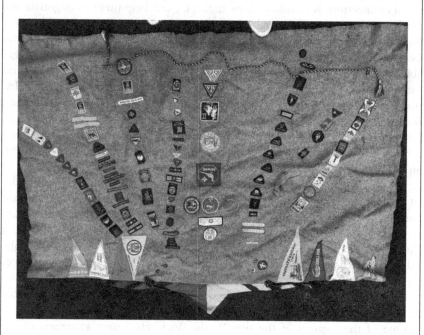

Figure 4.2 Camp blankets are a reminder of many scouting moments and achievements over the years

Source: Photograph by Julia Findon.

even the quietist will join in – although in the darkness it's generally easier to let go of one's inhibitions. But participation is entirely a matter of choice – no one is made to 'perform' if they would prefer not to.

At a smaller gathering there may be some 'skits'. These are short play-lets, which have been rehearsed beforehand. They are supposed to be funny, usually involving slapstick where someone may get wet or covered in soot. Once again, care is needed when picking someone as the butt of the joke, to avoid causing unnecessary embarrassment.

As the evening draws to a close, the singing ends with a quiet song to calm the high spirits, followed by a hot cup of cocoa before bed for the younger members. There is then the chance for the older scouts and leaders to sit around the fire chatting and reflecting on the day while watching the dying embers . . . a therapeutic end to the day, which will often remain a fond memory for many years to come.

Playful healing

When children encounter a seriously difficult life event, such as a major illness or an injury, the loss of a loved one, or a natural disaster, the quality of their social connections is critical to how their play can help them to negotiate the challenge to their psychosocial equilibrium. Linn (2008) reminds us that play flourishes in a community of caring adults who provide children with the essential gifts of time, space, and silence. Serious stress can be made more toler-able by the simple presence of loving adults who help the child to adapt and thrive through the modeling of positive coping behaviors. In times of difficulty, play becomes a comfort blanket, a distraction, and a release valve facilitating the restorative process of adaptation. The child with a rich play history has the potential to draw on learning from their bank of play experiences to overcome serious obstacles in ways that enhance, rather than compromise, their health and development (Fearn and Howard 2012).

When a child experiences frequent, prolonged, or uncontrollable episodes of adversity, such as extreme poverty, neglect, or repeated abuse, the associated stress becomes toxic with the potential to seriously disrupt developing brain circuits (National Scientific Council on the Developing Child 2015). No child should be expected to tolerate or adapt to toxic stress; it is now well estab-lished that toxic levels of stress in childhood can have lifelong consequences for the individual's physical and mental health (*ibid.*). Yet research also shows that developmental damage is not inevitable and that children can and do grow through the harshest of circumstances (Chatterjee 2018).

One of the legacies of the two World Wars was a new awareness of the impact of early trauma on childhood health and development. By the middle of the twentieth century, there was a growing recognition that children were vulnerable to experiential 'wounds to the spirit' (McCarthy 2014), and that separation from home and family through wartime evacuation, displacement, and bereavement had far-reaching consequences, both for the individual and for the wider social order (Shapira 2013). This realization fostered a cultural shift in understanding which recognized children's health and development as a reflection of the social milieu, and harm prevention became a public health priority in the decades following the Second World War (*ibid.*).

The British pediatrician and child psychologist Margaret Lowenfeld (1890–1973) was a pioneer in the use of 'play for healing' during the interwar years, making the case for play as a sensory language through which children might better share their feelings in relation to their life experiences, rather than by using spoken words (Lowenfeld 1991). Lowenfeld was a contemporary of Donald Winnicott (1896–1971), who also promoted play as a means of connecting the inner and outer world of the child. Winnicott regarded relationships as central to healthy development and coined the term 'potential space' to describe the safe, permissive, interpersonal field within which a person can be spontaneously playful while at the same time connected to others (Winnicott 1971: 106).

Box 4.6 The Island: non-directive play therapy with a bereaved sibling

Elizabeth Wilkinson

The World Technique (Lowenfeld 2011) is a way of engaging children in a therapeutic process which allows them to express themselves nonverbally through play. The therapist invites the child to build a picture of their world using wet and dry sand and a selection of representational objects and figures, explaining that the 'sand play' can help to express ideas and feelings which cannot be put into words.

The following account summarizes the use of the technique with Jenny (a pseudonym), aged nine years, following the death eighteen months previously of a brother two years her junior with whom she had a close sibling bond. She was referred for therapy having become withdrawn and solitary since the bereavement, avoiding interaction with a surviving sibling and struggling at school. She had previously resisted engagement with formal counseling. At the time of referral, the mother was newly pregnant, and Jenny had asked if the new baby was also going to die.

Jenny attended ten play therapy sessions over the course of twelve weeks, during which she engaged enthusiastically with this nondirective approach. Each session, Jenny meticulously arranged her sand tray and was adamant that no one else should touch it, insisting that her 'world' remain intact between sessions.

Jenny initially dug a grave at one end of the sand tray, complete with cross and gravestone. Toy figures (which she identified as her parents and herself) were placed at the opposite end of the tray. Invited to tell the story of her first tray, she explained that this was her brother's 'grave' and that the figures were the family standing near the grave 'missing him'. Although she was very chatty as she worked on subsequent trays, Jenny rarely referred again to her brother or spoke of any issues relating to his death.

Each week, Jenny would make small adjustments to her sand tray and then spend ten to fifteen minutes talking about it. Gradually, she spoke more openly about her feelings and about relationships in the family, themes which were reflected in changes made to the layout of the tray. On one occasion, she talked at length about her surviving sibling and the following week selected a toy to represent him, which she placed beside the other figures in the sand. In a later session, she talked about the impending arrival of the new baby in the family and placed the figure of 'a baby' alongside the rest of the family. She described them as 'all missing my brother'.

Over the following sessions, Jenny started to create a physical separation between 'the grave' and 'the family' in the sand tray. The distance between them increased week by week until eventually 'the grave' became 'an island' standing on its own. During the last two therapy sessions, Jenny asked for water to make 'a river', further isolating 'the island' and 'the grave' from 'the family' of figures. When satisfied with her final tray, she announced: 'Finished!' and when invited to talk about it, Jenny pointed to 'the island' and said, 'This is my brother's grave and (pointing to the figures) this is my family playing on the beach'. Her work was indeed 'finished'.

The World Technique reaches a deeper level of consciousness in the child and using the sand tray each week helped Jenny to organize her thoughts and literally 'play out' her feelings around the loss of her brother and the arrival of a new sibling. Having a visual image to reflect on at the end of each session helped her to develop a narrative about the issues which were impacting on her emotional growth and development. During the course of therapy, Jenny became closer to her younger sibling and enthusiastic about the new baby. She started to enjoy school again and her schoolwork improved.

In play therapy, Jenny had learned to understand her feelings, to cope with them, and control them. She had discovered that 'feelings can twist and turn and lose their sharp edges' (Axline 1964). The opportunity to play with feelings, which were previously beyond her grasp, allowed this child to grow through her grief toward a new level of personal and social resilience.

It was in the postwar climate of professional and public enlightenment regarding the impact of early experience on children's health that Susan Harvey, advisor to Save the Children Fund, drew attention to the trauma experienced by children in hospital. Referring to their separation from family, and the constraints of the hospital environment, she famously proclaimed that, 'Deprived of play, the child is a prisoner, shut off from all that makes life real and meaningful' (Harvey and Hales-Tooke 1972: 22). Harvey orchestrated the launch of the first hospital play scheme at the Brook Hospital in London in 1963 and was instrumental in setting up the first training course for Hospital Play Specialists which followed in 1973 (Jun Tai 2008).

Over the course of the past 50 years, the endorsement of therapeutic play and play-based services has enriched the healthcare experience of children, young people, and their families in the UK (National Association of Health Play Specialists n.d.) and around the globe (Association of Child Life Professionals 2017). Numerous studies testify to the benefits of therapeutic play for children in hospital in terms of establishing trust (Pan et al. 2004); assessing psychosocial needs (O'Connor and Drennan 2003); and reducing negative emotional behaviors (Ribeiro 2001), all of which are summarized in a policy statement on Child Life Services issued by the American Academy of Pediatrics (2014). Play and recreational activity are now widely regarded as essential to the provision of 'the best healthcare possible', advocated in Articles 24 and 31 of the United Nations Convention on the Rights of the Child (Tonkin 2014).

Box 4.7 Play is medicine too. A visit to the emergency department

Julia Whitaker

Loud screams herald the arrival of seven-year-old Sam in the Emergency Department, a blood-soaked towel clamped to his head. He is visibly terrified: wide-eyed, rigid, and clinging desperately to his mother. The pediatric assessment unit is designed such that new arrivals are steered past a play area before reaching the nurses' station, creating a bridge between the familiar world of home and the alien hospital environment. Passing the play area, Sam's screams subside as his attention is drawn to a familiar character in one of the toy boxes:

'Look Mum! They even have Thomas the Tank Engine here!'

The observant Health Play Specialist brings the toy train to meet Sam, initiating a friendly conversation about this popular children's character. She shows Sam that the toy engine also has a 'bump on the head' and suggests they both get checked over by 'the chief engineer'. The play specialist recognizes and accepts the developmental regression that frequently accompanies distress in the child; she knows that the use of his vivid imagination will be Sam's greatest asset as he undergoes assessment and treatment of his head injury, and thus begins the co-creation of a therapeutic play-story.

Sam is asked to clean Thomas's imaginary 'wound' while the nurse attends to his own and he engages in the play without question. The play specialist is aware that the magical thinking of the young child means that Sam might interpret his injury as a punishment for some misdemeanor, so she offers reassurance to the toy engine that he is not to blame for his damage, that he isn't in trouble for 'going off the rails'.

Sam listens attentively and strokes the toy, then asks what they will use to mend the engine. This is a cue for the play specialist to explain the procedure for closing Sam's own head wound, demonstrating on the toy engine and engaging Sam's help with the 'toolbox' of medical instruments. Lowenfeld (1991) described the child as 'thinking with his hands' and the play specialist knows that words alone offer inadequate explanation to the young child. She does not conceal that there will be some discomfort and shows the toy engine how he can 'puff out steam' to get rid of any painful feelings.

It is important that Sam remains still while his wound is closed and dressed, so the play specialist suggests a 'game' in which Sam and Thomas compete to see who can 'stay on the track' the longest. The treatment process is completed promptly, efficiently, and without any fuss, and Sam emerges intact from this threat to his physical and psychological integrity, with a renewed sense of self and of his personal resourcefulness.

The value of this play episode is reinforced by reference to Winnicott (1971: 54): 'It is in playing, and only in playing, that the individual child or adult is able to be creative and to use the whole personality, and it is only in being creative that the individual discovers the self'. The Health Play Specialist uses her knowledge of child development and her ability to swiftly establish rapport with the child to create 'a space for play' between imaginary possibility and external reality, akin to Winnicott's concept of potential space: 'a state of just being where identity can be suspended in creative play, in the absorbed exploration of potential' (Metcalfe and Game 2008).

Learning from the postwar period in Britain is now being extended to work with refugee children in Europe and Asia, where nongovernmental organizations are creating opportunities for play and creative self-expression through the arts as a route to healing from the horrors of present-day conflict and its consequences (e.g., Warner 2019).

The *Stories in Transit* project (Warner 2019), established in Palermo in Sicily in 2016, recognizes the rights of all people to cultural expression by encouraging migrants from Africa and the Middle East to share their stories using their own cultural traditions and imagination and enriching their narratives with a medley of creative media – art, music, puppetry, and games. Amidst the physical and emotional poverty of displacement, play comes to represent a place of safety and belonging: 'a collective self-protecting mechanism that thrives when children can create momentary time/space within their daily lives' (Lester and Russell 2014: 255).

In 2016, BRAC and the LEGO Foundation embarked on a partnership project to support play-based early childhood education in Bangladesh, Tanzania, and Uganda (BRAC 2016) based on the premise that: 'Our world is our playground, a platform for the creativity of all seven billion of us' (BRAC n.d.). Three years later, BRAC's Humanitarian Play Labs model is 'repurposing the Science of Play for settings troubled by humanitarian crisis' (Mariam cited in BRAC 2019), recognizing the healing power of play by creating safe spaces, reviving and nurturing children's natural spontaneity, and preserving a sense of cultural identity (Mariam and Saltmarsh 2019). It is through their play that children acquire the cultural values, skills, and abilities which nurture a sense of belonging and which anchor them in time and space.

Building resilience in a digital world

All the research into childhood resilience identifies the same two key factors for helping children to deal with challenge and adversity: access to a trusted adult (e.g., Bellis 2018), and access to play (e.g., Ginsburg and Jablow 2015). In the words of writer and childhood campaigner, Sue Palmer (2016: 70), 'the two key drivers of healthy development have always been parental love and children's freedom to play'. However, in the digital world of the twenty-first century, these two essential components of healthy child development are up against stiff competition from the seductive appeal of screens, smartphones, and other digital devices.

Research into the influence of digital technology on children's play and learning is a growing field of study (Internet.org 2020). A recent report by The LEGO Foundation (2018), for example, provides compelling evidence that digital play can engage children in knowledge and skills development, enhancing creativity and reinforcing social relationships. The use of digital technology has become integral to the social fabric worldwide, but this has raised parallel concerns that increased reliance on technology belies the challenges and dangers it poses to children's health and wellbeing (Center for Humane Technology 2019). While children's brains are still developing, they are vulnerable to being shaped by technology across a number of domains including: sleep patterns, nutrition, and the likelihood of obesity (Stiglic and Viner 2019); relationships (e.g., Uhis et al. 2014); and exposure to health-risk behaviors (e.g., Winpenny et al. 2014). Children living with cognitive challenges, or social challenges such as bullying and body image issues, may be especially vulnerable to the impact of technology use (van Geel et al. 2014) further exacerbating social disparities in health and wellbeing.

Taking into account the scientific evidence, the World Health Organization (WHO 2019) and the American Academy of Pediatrics (2016) advise a veto on screen-based activity under two years of age, no more than one hour a day between two and five years and a maximum of two hours a day thereafter until children reach double figures. In an article in the *Guardian* entitled 'Screen time v play time: what tech leaders won't let their own kids do', Fleming (2015) discusses the popularity among tech executives of Steiner-Waldorf schooling for their own offspring. The choice of Waldorf schools, which discourage the use of screens below 12 years of age, points to an even more cautionary approach to screen use for younger children.

In the UK, children engage in an average five hours of screen time per week, ranking fourth highest after the US, Denmark, and Saudi Arabia (The LEGO Foundation 2018). Yet despite this, 68 per cent of British children still say that they prefer to play with their friends face to face, compared with 25 per cent who prefer shared play online (*ibid.*). The LEGO report uses the term 'fluid play' to describe the overlap between the real world, the imagination, and digital experiences in the lives of children growing up in the twenty-first century. It emphasizes the role of parents in shaping their children's play, balancing screen time with other forms of play and taking an active part in the play. A study by Orth (2018), for example, found that when parents watch television with their children, they are more likely to learn new words, and test higher on cognitive abilities, than if they watch alone, suggesting that parental engagement can positively transform the impact of screen time.

When children are engaged in sedentary screen watching, they are missing out on both the resilience-building play behaviors outlined in Table 4.1 and the all-important face-to-face interactions with parents and peers. For school-aged children, screen time disrupts the development of healthy play behaviors because it decreases their ability to imagine the world, the development of the so-called mental imagery skills (BBC 2020). A child who is playing a digital game, or fixated on a television screen, is missing out on the physical and psychological benefits of real-life play experiences; and a child – or parent – who is glued to their phone is missing out on the close connection of an authentic relationship based on trust and unconditional love. The longer we can postpone the introduction of screen media into the lives of children, the bigger the window they have for creative play and for developing the skills and attributes that will prevent their dependence on it (Linn 2008). Dr Juana Willumsen (cited in World Health Organization 2019) puts it simply: 'What we really need to do is bring back [real] play for children'.

Conclusion

The school years see many significant changes in both the growing child's brain and in their experience of life and these are reflected in their play. During middle childhood, there is a divergence in the expression of gendered traits but a collective move toward greater independence of thought and behavior. As children continue to explore the world and their place in it, they need opportunities to take risks and to use the gift of their imagination to devise strategies for managing the challenges they face in life. As societies become more aware of the lifelong impact of adverse childhood experiences, there is a recognition that play, coupled with loving attention, is essential to the development of the skills and attributes that contribute to sustained resiliency, overall competence, and recovery from adversity (Brown 2019).

References

Administration for Children and Families (2019) *Head Start Programs*. Online. HTTP: <www.acf.hhs.gov/ohs/about/head-start> (accessed 2 June 2020).

American Academy of Pediatrics (2014) Policy statement: Child life services. *Pediatrics*, 133 (5): e1471–e1478.

American Academy of Pediatrics (2016) Policy statement: Media and young minds. *Pediatrics*, 138 (5): e20162591. https://doi.org/10.1542/peds.2016-2591.

Association of Child Life Professionals (2017) *The Need for Child Life Services*. Online. HTTP: <www.childlife.org/the-child-life-profession/the-case-for-child-life> (accessed 20 November 2020).

Axline, V. (1964) *Dibs in Search of Self*. New York: Houghton Mifflin.

BBC (2020) *Why the Way Our Children Watch Screens Matter*. Online. HTTP: <www.bbc.com/reel/video/p08k84jw/why-the-way-our-children-watch-screens-matters> (accessed 17 August 2020).

Bellis, M. A., Hughes, K., Ford, K., Hardcastle, K., Sharp, A., Wood, S., Homolova, L. and Davies, A. (2018) Adverse childhood experiences and sources of childhood resilience: A retrospective study of their combined relationships with child health and educational attendance. *BMC Public Health*, 18: 792. doi.org/10.1186/s12889-018-5699-8.

Börnert-Ringleb, M. and Wilbert, J. (2018) The Association of Strategy Use and Concrete-Operational Thinking in Primary School. *Frontiers in Education*, 3 (38). Online. HTTP: <https://doi.org/10.3389/feduc.2018.00038> (accessed 20 July 2020).

Boyd, H. and Bee, D. (2012) *The Developing Child*. 13th ed. New York: Pearson Education, Inc.

BRAC (2016) *BRAC and the LEGO Foundation Collaborate on Play-to-Learn Project*. Online. HTTP: <www.brac.net/latest-news/item/940-brac-and-the-lego-foundation-collaborate-on-play-to-learn-project> (accessed 23 May 2020).

BRAC (2019) *Humanitarian Play Labs: Helping Rohingya Children Heal and Learn through Play*. Online. HTTP: <www.brac.net/latest-news/item/1213-humanitarian-play-labs-helping-rohingya-children-heal-and-learn-through-play> (accessed 23 May 2020).

BRAC (n.d.) *Who We Are*. Online. HTTP: <www.brac.net/who-we-are> (accessed 23 May 2020).

Brizendine, L. (2007) *The Female Brain*. New York: Bantam Books.

Brizendine, L. (2011) *The Male Brain: An Essential Owner's Manual for Every Man, and a Cheat Sheet for Every Woman*. New York: Bantam Books.

Brown, S. (2008) *Play Is More Than Just Fun*. Online. HTTP: <www.ted.com/talks/stuart_brown_play_is_more_than_just_fun?language=en> (accessed 7 October 2020).

Brown, S. (2019) *The Science of Play: How Play Helps Us Develop Resilience*. Online. HTTP: <www.playcore.com/news/how-play-helps-us-develop-resilience> (accessed 18 July 2020).

Care (2020) *Girls' Education*. Online. HTTP: <www.care.org/work/education/girls-education> (accessed 29 April 2020).

Center for Humane Technology (2019) *Home*. Online. HTTP: <https://humanetech.com/>.

Chatterjee, S. (2018) Unleashing the power of play: Research from the International Play Association 20th Triennial Conference. *Children, Youth and Environments*, 28 (2): 119–145.

City, University of London (2017) *Toy Story: New Study Looks into How Gender Toy Preferences Have Changed since the 80s*. Online. HTTP: <www.city.ac.uk/news/2017/november/toy-story-new-study-looks-into-how-gender-toy-preferences-have-changed-since-the-80s#:~:text=From%20an%20early%20age%2C%20children,of%20methods%20and%20social%20contexts> (accessed 15 July 2020).

Cornelissen, T. and Dustmann, C. (2019) *The Benefits of Starting School Early*. Online. HTTP: <https://voxeu.org/article/benefits-starting-school-early> (accessed 2 June 2020).

DelGiudice, M. (2017) Middle childhood: An evolutionary-developmental synthesis. In: Halfon, N., Forrest, C., Lerner, R. and Faustman, E. (Eds.), *Handbook of Life Course Health Development*: 95–107. New York: Springer.

Dent, M. (2003) *Saving Our Children from Our Chaotic World: Teaching Children the Magic of Silence and Stillness*. Murwillumbah, Australia: Pennington Publications.

DK (2006) *A Life Like Mine: How Children Live around the World*. London: Dorling Kindersley.

Egan, K. and Judson, G. (2015) *Imagination and the Engaged Learner: Cognitive Tools for the Classroom*. New York: Teachers College Press.

Fearn, M. and Howard, J. (2012) Play as a resource for children facing adversity: An exploration of indicative case studies. *Children and Society*, 26: 456–468.

Fleming, A. (2015) Screen Time v Play Time: What Tech Leaders Won't Let Their Own Kids Do. Online. HTTP: <www.theguardian.com/technology/2015/may/23/screen-time-v-play-time-what-tech-leaders-wont-let-their-own-kids-do> (accessed 20 November 2020).

Ginsburg, K. R. and Jablow, M. M. (2015) *Building Resilience in Children and Teens: Giving Kids Roots and Wings*. 3rd ed. Elk Grove Village, IL: American Academy of Pediatrics.

Gray, P. (2008) *A Brief History of Education: To Understand Schools, We Must View Them in Historical Perspective*. Online. HTTP: <www.psychologytoday.com/gb/blog/freedom-learn/200808/brief-history-education> (accessed 29 April 2020).

Harvey, S. and Hales-Tooke, A. (Eds.) (1972) *Play in Hospital*. London: Faber.

International Play Association [IPA] (2020) *UN Convention on the Rights of the Child*. Online. HTTP: <http://ipaworld.org/childs-right-to-play/uncrc-article-31/un-convention-on-the-rights-of-the-child-1/> (accessed 2 June 2020).

Internet.org (2020) *Discovering Digital at Primary*. Online. HTTP: <www.internetmatters.org/resources/discovering-digital-at-primary-school/> (accessed 18 July 2020).

Joel, D. and Vikhanski, L. (2019) *Gender Mosaic: Beyond the Myth of the Male and Female Brain*. Boston, MA: Little, Brown.

Jun Tai, N. (2008) Play in hospital. *Therapeutic Play Journal*. Online. HTTP: <www.thetcj.org/in-residence/play-in-hospital> (accessed 16 January 2020).

Krampen, M. (2013) *Children's Drawings: Iconic Coding of the Environment*. Berlin: Springer Science & Business Media.

Landreth, G. (2002) *Play Therapy: The Art of the Relationship*. New York: Brunner Routledge.

The LEGO Foundation (2018) *LEGO Play Well Report 2018*. Online. HTTP: <www.legofoundation.com/media/1441/lego-play-well-report-2018.pdf> (accessed 4 May 2020).

Lester, S. and Russell, W. (2008) *Play for a Change: Play, Policy and Practice: A Review of Contemporary Perspectives*. London: National Children's Bureau.

Lester, S. and Russell, W. (2014) Turning the world upside down: Playing as the deliberate creation of uncertainty. *Children*, 1: 241–260.

Linn, S. (2008) *The Case for Make Believe: Saving Play in a Commercialized World*. New York: The New Press.

Lowenfeld, M. (1991) *Play in Childhood*. Cambridge: Cambridge University Press.

Lowenfeld, M. (2011) *Understanding Children's Sandplay: Lowenfeld's World Technique*. Eastbourne, UK: Sussex Academic Press.

Ludicology (2020, 1 July) *Play Sufficiency: A Population Health Priority*. [Blog]. Online. HTTP: <https://ludicology.com/store-room/play-sufficiency-a-population-health-priority/> (accessed 13 July 2020).

Lukianoff, G. and Haidt, J. (2018) *The Coddling of the American Mind: How Good Intentions and Bad Ideas Are Setting Up a Generation for Failure*. New York: Penguin.

Mah, V. K. and Ford-Jones, E. L. (2012) Spotlight on middle childhood: Rejuvenating the 'forgotten years'. *Paediatrics and Child Health*, 17 (2): 81–83.

Mariam, E. and Saltmarsh, S. J. (2019) *Can Play Save a Displaced Generation?* Online. HTTP: <www.brac.net/publications/dbrief/can-play-save-a-displaced-generation/> (accessed 23 May 2020).

McCarthy, H. (2014) Review of *The War Inside: Psychoanalysis, Total War and the Making of the Democratic Self in Post-War Britain* (review no. 1600). Reviews in History. Online. HTTP: <https://reviews.history.ac.uk/review/1600> (accessed 13 January 2020).

McCarthy, M. (2016) Sex differences in the developing brain as a source of inherent risk. *Dialogues in Clinical Neuroscience*, 18 (4): 361–372.

Metcalfe, A. and Game, A. (2008) Potential space and love. *Emotion, Space and Society*, 1 (1): 18–21.

Ministry of Children and Youth Services (2017) *On My Way: A Guide to Support Middle Years Development*. Toronto: Ministry of Children and Youth Services.

National Association of Health Play Specialists (n.d.) *NAHPS Milestones*. Online. HTTP: <www.nahps.org.uk/> (accessed 20 November 2020).

National Scientific Council on the Developing Child (2015) *Supportive Relationships and Active Skill-Building Strengthen the Foundations of Resilience*. Working Paper 13. Cambridge, MA: Center on the Developing Child, Harvard University.

Nicholson, J., Shimpi, P. M. and Rabin, P. (2013) 'If I am not doing my own playing then I am not able to truly share the gift of play with children': Using poststructuralism and care ethics to examine future early childhood educators' relationships with play in adulthood. *Early Child Development and Care*, 184 (8): 1192–1210. doi.org/10.1080/03004430. 2013.856894.

O'Connor, G. and Drennan, C. (2003) Optimising patient care: Meeting the needs of the paediatric oncology patient. *Journal of Diagnostic Radiography and Imaging*, 5: 33–38.

Openlearn (2016) *Curriculum Frameworks and Play*. Online. HTTP: <www.open.edu/openlearn/education/professional-development-education/the-role-play-childrens-learning/content-section-1.1> (accessed 14 July 2020).

Orth, U. (2018) The family environment in early childhood has a long-term effect on self-esteem: A longitudinal study from birth to age 27 years. *Journal of Personality and Social Psychology*, 114 (2): 637–655.

Palmer, S. (2016) *Upstart: The Case for Raising the School Starting Age and Providing What the Under-Sevens Really Need*. Edinburgh: Floris Books.

Pan, H., Chiu, P., Shen, J. and Chen, C. (2004) Application of therapeutic play in the process of nursing a preschool patient. *Hu LI Za Zhi [Journal of Nursing]*, 51: 94–100.

PBS Education (2020) *How We Can Bring Creativity and Imagination Back to the Classroom*. Online. HTTP: <www.pbs.org/education/blog/how-we-can-bring-creativity-and-imagination-back-to-the-classroom> (accessed 9 July 2020).

Pearson, E., Umayahara, M. and Ndijuye, L. (2017) *Play and Resilience*. Online. HTTP: <https://docplayer.net/86520958-Supporting-childhood-resilience-through-play-a-facilitation-guide-for-early-childhood-practitioners.html> (accessed 17 January 2021).

Ribeiro, P. J., Sabates, A. L. and Ribeiro, C. A. (2001) The use of a therapeutic toy as an instrument of nursing intervention when preparing the child to blood collection. *Revista da Escola de Enfermagem da USP*, 35: 420–428.

Rutter, M. (1985) Resilience in the face of adversity: Protective factors and resistance to psychiatric disorder. *British Journal of Psychiatry*, 147: 598–611.

Shakespeare, W. (2006) *As You Like It*. 3rd Series. London: The Arden Shakespeare.

Shapira, M. (2013) *The War Inside: Psychoanalysis, Total War and the Making of the Democratic Self in Post-War Britain*. Cambridge: Cambridge University Press.

Stiglic, N. and Viner, R. M. (2019) Effects of screentime on the health and well-being of children and adolescents: A systematic review of reviews. *BMJ Open*, 9: e023191. doi:10.1136/ bmjopen-2018-023191.

Sugar Lake Lodge (2020, 6 May) *The Power of Campfires: The Original Social Network*. [Blog]. Online. HTTP: <https://sugarlakelodge.com/blog/power-of-campfires/> (accessed 14 July 2020).

Sutton-Smith, B. (2008) Play theory: A personal journey and new thoughts. *American Journal of Play*, Summer: 80–123.

Take Care Staff (2018) *Boys' and Girls' Brains: Similar to Start, Changed by Environment*. Online. HTTP: <www.wrvo.org/post/boys-and-girls-brains-similar-start-changed-environment#stream/0> (accessed 19 November 2020).

Todd, B. K., Fischer, R. A., Di Costa, S., Roestorf, A., Harbour, K., Hardiman, P. and Barry, J. (2017) Sex differences in children's toy preferences: A systematic review, meta-regression, and meta-analysis. *Infant and Child Development*, 27 (2): e2064. doi. org/10.1002/icd.2064.

Tonkin, A. (2014) *The Provision of Play in Health Service Delivery: Fulfilling Children's Rights under Article 31 of the United Nations Convention on the Rights of the Child: A Literatrue Review*. Online. HTTP: <www.england.nhs.uk/6cs/wp-content/uploads/sites/25/2015/03/nahps-full-report.pdf> (accessed 19 November 2020).

Too Much Too Soon (n.d.) *UK Children Deserve Something Better*. Online. HTTP: <www.toomuchtoosoon.org/> (accessed 29 April 2020).

Uhis, Y. T., Michikyan, M., Morris, J., Garcia, D., Small, G., Zgourou, E. and Greenfiled, P. (2014) Five days at outdoor education camp without screens improves preteen skills with nonverbal emotion cues. *Computers in Human Behavior*, 39: 387–392.

UNICEF (2020) *Convention on the Rights of the Child Text*. Online. HTTP: <www.unicef.org/child-rights-convention/convention-text> (accessed 14 July 2020).

Upstart (n.d.) *Reasons for Upstart: Why Do We Need a Kindergarten Stage*. Online. HTTP: <www.upstart.scot/reasons/> (accessed 29 April 2020).

van Geel, M., Vedder, P. and Tanilon, J. (2014) Relationship between peer victimization, cyberbullying, and suicide in children and adolescents: A meta-analysis. *JAMA Pediatrics*, 168 (5): 435–442.

Warner, M. (2019) Living in a country of words: The shelter of stories. In: Fernyhough, C. (Ed.), *Others*. London: Unbound: 233–251.

Winnicott, D. (1971) *Playing and Reality*. London: Penguin.

Winpenny, E. M., Marteau, T. M. and Nolte, E. (2014) Exposure of children and adolescents to alcohol marketing on social media websites. *Alcohol*, 49 (2): 154–159.

World Health Organization (2019) *To Grow Up Healthy, Children Need to Sit Less and Play More*. Online. HTTP: <www.who.int/news-room/detail/24-04-2019-to-grow-up-healthy-children-need-to-sit-less-and-play-more> (accessed 2 May 2020).

Zhang, X. Y., DeBlois, L., Deniger, M. A. and Kamanzi, C. (2008) A theory of success for disadvantaged children: Reconceptualization of social capital in the light of resilience. *Alberta Journal of Educational Research*, 54 (1): 97–111.

5 Adolescence

According to Arain et al. (2013: 449) 'adolescence is the developmental epoch during which children become adults – intellectually, physically, hormonally, and socially . . . full of changes and transformations'. Nowhere is this more evident than in the brain. With advances in Magnetic Resonance Imaging (MRI) over the past 25 years, functionality and regional morphology have become evident (Arian et al. 2013) which indicates that the teenage brain is not yet ready or able to work in the same way as that of adults (Paediatric Society of New Zealand 2020). This knowledge allows us, as the wider community, to anticipate and mitigate for the 'dramatic re-configuration that occurs' during this stage (Carter 2018: 24). The developing adolescent brain needs 'a safe environment where they have consistent, loving support . . . clear, consistent boundaries, and very importantly, their growing capacity and ability to do things independently needs to be respected' (Paediatric Society of New Zealand 2020). More than simply a stage to get over, adolescence is 'a stage of life to cultivate well' (Siegel 2014).

The adolescent phase of brain development is characterized by a second wave of synaptogenesis, leading to major maturational change which stabilizes around 25 years of age (Carter 2018). Synaptogenesis is 'a long developmental process involving synapse formation, synapse maintenance (stabilization), and activity-dependent synapse refinement and elimination, and is important for the establishment of the neuronal network and the precision of brain circuitry' (Cohen-Cory, cited in Science Direct 2020). The brain matures from back to front and, by the time children reach puberty, the back of the brain, which is responsible for perception, has generally matured (Carter 2018). At this point, the brain undergoes a 're-wiring process' which lasts throughout adolescence, as the pruning of dendrites eliminates unused synapses and myelination increases the speed of impulse conduction (Arian et al. 2013). This is particularly prevalent in the prefrontal cortex, where the brain makes and remakes neural connections at a phenomenal rate (Carter 2018: 24), resulting in region-specific vulnerability due to the continuous reconstruction and maturation of the neurocircuitry (Arian et al. 2013). As a result of this exceptional brain plasticity, this sensitive period of brain development allows for the acquisition of new learning and skills and opportunities for forging lifelong interests and talents (Arian et al. 2013). This second period of rapid synaptogenesis means that the kind of environmental stimuli available to teenagers will literally shape their brain structure, reinforcing the vital importance of this developmental stage for lifelong health and potential.

With all the cognitive, social, emotional, behavioral, and physical changes that occur during adolescence, it can be easy to forget that teenagers still need opportunities to play and that they seek fun and friendship just as much as they did in earlier developmental phases (Make Time 2 Play 2020). In adolescence, play is devoted to exploring and developing a personal identity and to finding one's place in the world (*ibid.*). Pat Kane (n.d.), advocating the concept of a *play ethic*, writes: 'First of all, don't take "play" to mean anything idle, wasteful of frivolous. This is "play" as the great philosophers understood it: the experience of being an active, creative and fully autonomous person'.

Young poet, Theresa Lola (cited in Douglas 2020a) underlines the serious nature of the adolescent's journey toward personhood: 'Identity isn't always a straightforward thing . . . There are so many different components to it and complex ways in which we view ourselves'. Self-expression through cultural art forms including poetry, art and music provides a creative outlet for the adolescent's playful experimentation with the idea of self and of community. Lola (*ibid.*) explains,

> There's hope in being able to share what you're going through and your view of the world. Poetry isn't just about writing things the way they are – we can also imagine the way we want things to be. There's something almost miraculous about that kind of act.

The following poem, by Sonny McLeod, demonstrates how poetry can articulate the playfulness which permeates a young person's thoughts and feelings, reminding us that open dialogue and opportunities for self-expression are essential for enabling young people to share their internal experiences in a way that feels both safe and satisfying (Make Time 2 Play 2020).

Box 5.1 We're all playing

Sonny G. C. McLeod

We're all playing

I like poetry, but I struggle finding the words, like birds they leave for a new world never to be controlled, they flow out.

Thinking up the pace, finding the room and space, it's one massive guessing game.

We're all playing. We all have ideas. They come one, two, three now I need tea but I can't one, two, three here they come too fast.

We're all playing, all waiting on the delaying till we're slamming, till we're clapping, clicking, tapping, awaiting our time and the words you next . . .

We're all playing, we're in this together, forever, till the clock hits quarter to eleven of the first of November.

Here I stand, throwing out words you may not understand, so now I think come on man get it together for this guessing game, we're in this together, we're all playing.

I like poetry, but even when I find the words, I just stutter, they all clutter together, I'm like fuck not again you can do better, you may not control the weather be capable of holding yourself together but you can write. Right or wrong the words still come, rhyme or not this is still pretty damn fun, is it not? Is it not a game, a maze to find the words to play with, and finding the courage to say them.

You clear your head, restarting the game instead of delaying it, creating your own board instead of playing the old.

It's our time to shine, our time to be fine, listen to each other's rhyme we've designed why?! Cause we're all playing.

Parents, passion, and purpose: what adolescents need

The prevailing perception of adolescence – fueled by popular culture and media stereotypes – is that it is a period of inevitable turmoil and rebellion and that teenagers are fundamentally different and disconnected from the rest of us. However, Aubrun and Grady (2000) remind us that, while the social and cultural context of adolescence changes over the course of history, young people essentially do not. Neither 'monsters' nor 'heroes', most teenagers are indeed 'regular people': responsible, hard-working, and highly moral, with mainstream views and interests (*ibid.*). Benson (2008: 40) goes further, describing teenagers as delightful, idealistic, exuberant, and creative, celebrating the potential of adolescence as a period of 'exploding into possibility'.

Despite a widely broadcast rise in mental health problems among adolescents, the truth is that most young people enjoy good physical and mental health (Mental Health Foundation 2020), and teenagers are more likely to be the victims than perpetrators of crime (Child Trends 2018). The trend for tattooing and body-piercing is followed only by a high-profile minority of teens (Breuner and Levine 2017), and the same is true for excessive drug and alcohol use (Office for National Statistics 2013). This is not to deny that there are a significant, and growing, minority of young people who need expert professional help for mental health or substance abuse problems – but these problems are not a function of their developmental stage (Kubik et al. 2019). The majority of adolescents report few or no symptoms of depression (Jewell et al. 2018) and longitudinal research shows that cigarette, alcohol, and illegal drug use has reduced over the course of several years (Johnston et al. 2016).

Siegel (2014) writes: 'Young minds are often portrayed as stews of hormones and impulse; but the decisions they make are often deeply rational and deserving of greater consideration'. While the baseline level of dopamine is lower during adolescence (Arain et al. 2013), its release in response to experience is higher (Siegel 2014), which both explains the teenage mood swings and also accounts for the creative energy and positive bias characteristic of the teenage years. Siegel (2014) proposes that the emotional spark, novelty-seeking, creative exploration, and social engagement associated with adolescence are necessary core aspects of this developmental stage which 'enable adolescents to develop vital new capacities that they can use to lead happier and healthier lives'.

When thinking about adolescent health and wellbeing it is, therefore, perhaps most useful to look at the majority of young people who are navigating this transitional stage with clear promise and purpose. Australian psychologist, Steve Biddulph (2013, 2015) has synthesized clinical experience and relevant research to come up with a prescription for a happy, healthy adolescence which recognizes the different needs of teenage boys and girls. This can be summarized as the adolescent's need for Parents, Passion, and Purpose.

Teens need parents

Biddulph (2017) challenges the widespread belief that children need their parents less as they grow older, suggesting instead that they need their parents more than ever in the teenage years. The interaction between the adolescent's natural drive for autonomy and a strong parental attachment is commonly portrayed as a conflictual tussle. However, research suggests that these apparently contradictory processes interrelate in complex ways which can help us to understand differences in psychosocial adjustment during the adolescent years (Boykin McElhaney et al. 2009).

A robust parent–adolescent attachment is important because it 'provides a secure base in which to understand, rehearse and manage the strong affect that might be associated with managing new relationships' (Shaw and Dallos 2005: 418). Recent research found that parental attachment was associated with more positive peer relationships and lower levels of both internalizing and externalizing problems (Jager et al. 2015). The quality of the attachment relationship is critical to how young people learn to cope with social and societal pressures, including commercial exploitation, peer pressure, and fashion and behavioral trends (Boykin McElhaney et al. 2009). Teenagers need a safe 'rehearsal space' within which to explore and experiment with different ideas and identities before they venture into the adult world and, for most young people, it is within the security of 'family' that they find this space. Philippa Perry (2020: 270) writes, 'Just like the stage your child went through when they were a toddler discovering their autonomy, teens need love plus boundaries and a heavy dose of parental optimism that they will master their emotions and their impulsivity'. During periods of adolescent uncertainty and self-questioning, it is 'parents [who] can provide extra scaffolding that helps them get through' (Dahl, cited in Suttie 2016).

Play has an important role in reinforcing attachment at developmental intersections because it can be a conduit for individuation within a close emotional relationship: a blueprint for successful peer and partner relationships in adulthood. Steinberg (2014: 134) attests that, 'adolescents appear to do best when they grow up in a family atmosphere that permits the development of individuality against a backdrop of close family ties'.

The dynamic nature of play means that it is a benign shapeshifter, changing with the developmental seasons, and families who make time and space for play can sustain emotional connection through periods of transition. Perry (2020: 276) reminds us that

> [I]t's important to spend time with our children whatever their age, and to listen to them, not only to be with them when we are all staring at separate screens, or living mostly separate lives and merely sharing a space. We need to make sure we connect with them as well as live with them.

Birthday and celebration rituals, shared interests and enthusiasms, time spent together in nature, and joint involvement in the wider community: all represent opportunities for continuing attachment play into adolescence. Having an attitude that anything can be fun means that the most mundane of everyday activities can be reframed as play (Whitaker 2019). It is not just the quality, but also the quantity, of time spent together that is important (Jewell et al. 2018): teens need both 'focused times and hang around times' with their parents (Galinsky 1999: 92).

Teens need a 'passion'

Biddulph (2013) is a strong advocate for intrinsically motivated activities as a way of keeping young people grounded throughout the hormonal fluctuations of the teenage years. Having a passion or 'spark' – be it for sport, music, dance, or a social cause – which is supported both from within and without the family, closely correlates with positive health and wellbeing in adolescence (Benson 2008). Getting involved with something that they 'love to do' enriches and strengthens the teenager because it not only nourishes their creative spirit but also provides an extended cross-generational reference group (Biddulph 2013). Teens need the feeling of belonging to a 'tribe' to support their wellbeing (*ibid.*) and real-world connections made through the sharing of passions and enthusiasms are healthier than those made in the anonymity of cyberspace.

Young people also need positive role-models, adults outside of the family, who are interested in them and enjoy their company; someone who inspires them to pursue their own goals and dreams and offers them a broader perspective on the world. During adolescence, the *nucleus accumbens*, the part of the limbic system linked to motivation and reward, becomes acutely sensitive

(Arain et al. 2013), which means that teenagers are more responsive to positive reinforcement than to criticism and sanctions (Paediatric Society of New Zealand 2020). Former England and Arsenal footballer, Ian Wright, pays tribute to his former teacher, Mr Pigden, who, rather than punishing him for misbehavior, taught him patience and confidence and so 'opened up the world to [him]', literally changing the course of his life (Speck 2018).

Biddulph (2013) advocates the adoption of such benevolent 'uncles' and 'aunties' as the modern equivalents of the community 'elders' who imparted wisdom and spiritual guidance in former times. Science affirms that that the availability of at least one stable, caring, and supportive relationship is key to developing resilience in life and, along with the competencies acquired through play, can transform toxic stress into something more manageable (National Scientific Council on the Developing Child 2015).

In his memoir, *My name Is Why* (2019), the author and broadcaster, Lemn Sissay (2019), recalls the teacher who gave him a copy of *The Mersey Sounds*, his first book of poems, and in doing so nourished his own literary aspirations. He also names the community worker, whose gift of a biography of Bob Marley represented a tangible acknowledgment of the internal distress Sissay shared with the famous musician. For young people who do not readily find older, supportive adults within their own social circle, the benevolent intervention of such an interested and attentive 'mentor' can have a positive impact on self-esteem and confidence in their own abilities (Schwartz et al. 2012).

The S.M.I.L.E-ing Boys Project (Douglas 2020b) inspired by artist Kai-Rufai adopts a playful approach to enabling young people to 'give voice' to their identity and to tell their own story. Drawing on the 8 Pillars of Happiness defined by the Happiness Research Institute (2020) in Copenhagen, Denmark, this research-led music, poetry, and immersive arts project provides young black boys growing up in London with a sense of agency over the factors that affect their future wellbeing – literally giving them something to smile about. Darnell (cited in universalsoulartist 2019), one of the participants in the S.M.I.L.E-ing Boys workshops says of his mentor:

> He's really a joyful guy, a guy I can really speak to. Since he came here, it's opened up my mind to so many things. It makes me want to wake up to the morning and see him speak. It's inspirational.

The capabilities that underlie resilience can be strengthened at any age (National Scientific Council on the Developing Child 2015). Engagement in age-appropriate activities which confer benefits to health, and which are undertaken in a culturally affirming context, improves the odds that a teen will thrive and will develop the capacities to cope with, adapt to, and even prevent adversity in their lives. The following case-story by Ike Odina exemplifies the role of the mentor–mentee relationship and how play provides a conduit through which young people can develop skills that will allow them to navigate their developmental path toward adulthood.

Box 5.2 When play works wonders: *Mentors Inspiratus . . . !!*

Ike C. Odina

Play is one of life's true 'freedom fighters', liberating us from life's 'musts, shoulds, and have to's'. Play has a wonderful ability to reveal and release one's authentic self; often hidden under layers of having to conform to/comply with (often) unfounded, yet deeply sedimented, stereotypes and social norms.

However, there seems to be an unspoken legend passing from one generation to the next which implies that, the further we grow away from childhood, the less we need to play. This flies in the face of the fact that most of today's so-called A-listers (actors, politicians, statesmen) make their living by 'playing' different roles . . . and continue to do so right up until their terminal breath. To paraphrase The Bard, *life is a stage and we are all players*. We all have our parts to play . . .

Mentors Inspiratus . . . !! is a not-for-profit mentoring group whose aim is to provide opportunities for young people to see the benefits of and ultimately choose to be good (global) citizens. We achieve our objective(s) by helping our mentees to identify themselves and their purpose and then encourage them to use their abilities to pursue this purpose. As a mentor of young people, I find that play enables our mentees to achieve greater heights and depths, than when we employ only the language of 'work'.

Our mentees are enrolled on our Young Leadership Program, which identifies five different types of leader – Visionaries, Ideas people, Planners, Builders, and Checkers – each of which embodies a different set of skills and abilities. All our mentees have been able to identify themselves (predominantly) with one of these leadership types and are regularly presented with opportunities to demonstrate, validate, nurture, and develop their unique abilities. For the past five years, I have had the pleasure of watching our mentees grow into even more delightful young people . . . than when I first met them.

Play is the perfect canvas on which our young leaders can present themselves to the world. In addition to regular play activities such as football, Swing-Ball, Chess, quizzes etc., we sometimes organize a day-out for fun and play. One of such favored events is our trip to the local wall-climbing center, where our mentees have up to three hours of unadulterated (interesting word – sometimes it takes an adult to complicate and mess things) play, followed by . . . pizza!

Despite my being their mentor, the young people allow – even *want* – me to join in with the play and it is wonderful to see their skills and innate abilities come alive during these times of play. More often than not, the Visionaries and the Planners have already come up with an action plan of what we do when we get to the Centre. The Builders and Checkers have a knack for sorting everybody out and implementing the agreed plan. At the end of all the fun, it is the skill of the Ideas people and Visionaries to take the lead and come up with ideas for future days out.

For *Mentors Inspiratus . . . !!* play is both the vehicle and the route by which our mentees become quite adept at navigating through life. The 'sense of play' simplifies matters and makes them much easier to deal with. In and through play, our mentees have discovered what they excel at and what others are brilliant at too. With this in mind, teamwork, delegation and ultimately the achievement of group objectives become that much easier.

Our innate ability to play, when given freedom of expression, reveals inner strengths and abilities, which might otherwise remain untapped. Let's learn to and get into the uplifting habit of playing as hard as we work.

Teens need to find a purpose

Damon et al. (2003) state that adolescence is 'a formative period for cultivating a sense of purpose', expressed in the desire and motivation 'to make a difference in the world, to contribute to matters larger than the self' (*ibid.*: 121). Seligman (2011) writes that wellbeing depends on increasing the amount of 'flourishing' in both one's own life and in the planet and it is noteworthy that the constituent features of flourishing – self-esteem, optimism, resilience, vitality, self-determination, and positive relationships – are also defining features of play. Play represents 'a refuge from ordinary life, a sanctuary of the mind' (Ackerman 1999: 6), and it is in the 'sacred place' of play, rather than through the satisfaction of primitive drives or selfish ambition, that the young person will find the purpose that gives meaning to their life.

When a young person has a sense of purpose, based on both a love of life and of the world, they become sufficiently well-centered to avoid the drift toward ideological extremes. In contrast, 'a youngster without a noble purpose may be like a vacuum that can be filled with unwholesome elements of all kinds' (Damon et al. 2003: 126). The value of a sense of purpose extends beyond the adolescent period, influencing health and wellbeing throughout the lifespan (Alimujiang et al. 2019). It may be that purpose acts as a buffer against stress and that 'having a global sense that life is meaningful and feeling that one matters in the world, has a purpose, and that life makes sense may be related to more adaptive coping skills' (Hooker et al. 2018).

Bernie de Koven (2013) introduced the concept of the 'well-played game' and its relationship to the well-lived life. In an interview in 2017, he explained: 'the well-played game has nothing to do with who wins or loses. It's all about how we play together. As such, it is a template, a model for a well-lived life' (De Koven 2017). The following case-story by Cristina illustrates how the discovery that we can play well together increases our ability to both embrace challenge and to seek out new challenges in life (*ibid.* 2013).

Box 5.3 Playing in the gap: meeting the challenge of self-discovery

Cristina Grohmann

I have always enjoyed traveling and exploring new places. I am fascinated by different cultures, languages, and ways of living – but I dislike being a tourist. Spending a short time somewhere, with little opportunity to really get to know a place, can only ever result in a superficial experience. So, when deciding what to do during my Gap Year, I chose not to backpack around Europe, but to spend the year in a single country doing something to help the local community. This would allow me to experience a whole new way of life in a truly immersive manner while doing something meaningful. This was the start of my journey with Project Trust (2020).

Project Trust is an educational charity that provides gap-year opportunities to school leavers, giving them the chance to live and work in a number of communities across the globe. Volunteers are selected over the course of four days on the Isle of Coll in the Inner Hebrides, where they are also trained before traveling overseas and then debriefed on their return. The selection course is intended to replicate the year abroad and designed, not just to assess prospective volunteers, but to allow them to discover whether they are sufficiently motivated to take on the challenge of a year doing something completely different.

The selection course was an opportunity for us to learn more about the charity and for them to learn about us through our participation in various games. Separated into groups to tackle assigned tasks, my fellow volunteers and myself first had to interpret the rules of the games. I don't want to ruin the experience for any future volunteers by disclosing details of the selection activities, but they demanded a willingness to embrace playful thinking. At first glance the activities seemed almost childish, but they were incredibly challenging, and I found them deeply meaningful. Even when we seemed to fail to achieve the intended outcome, we found we had inadvertently made good friends with one another in the process of trying.

Some of our afternoons on Coll were dedicated to outdoor work helping the island community and one day, during a gap in the timetable, we initiated an impromptu game of hide-and-seek. Together with some members of the staff team, we found ourselves ducking beneath old stone walls and hiding behind boulders in the heather, our hearts beating wildly at the sound of approaching footsteps. Any social anxiety which might have previously restricted our behavior soon disappeared and back came the childish excitement at the prospect of being the last one caught.

Our time on the island was rounded off with a ceilidh: a mismatched group of dancers, some well versed in the art of ceilidh-dancing and others learning the steps for the first time. Once again, inhibitions fell away as we whirled round the room to the accelerating fiddle music. Such a carefree feeling of freedom and confidence was something that I recognized from those unrehearsed moments when the rest of the world fades into the background and what is left is the excitement and the satisfaction of joining the game in hand.

Playful learning in adolescence

One of the downsides of recent educational reform has been 'the erosion of creativity, play and joy' in the day-to-day lives of teenagers (Conklin 2015). Research shows that the decline in opportunities for play since the 1950s has been paralleled by the widely reported increase in mental health problems among young people (Gray 2011). Kasser (2002) makes the link between anxiety and depression and a focus on extrinsic goals over intrinsic goals in the experience of young people. Extrinsic goals are those motivated by the values of others (exam grades, status, money, 'looking good') while intrinsic goals are derived from self-motivated pursuits such as the mastery of an activity one enjoys, making friends, pursuing a cause, and finding meaning in life. Since play is the enactment of intrinsic motivation, it is reasonable to conclude that the decline in play may be the factor that has most directly contributed to the decline in young people's mental health (Gray 2011).

The following case-story describes the use of play to transform the classroom experience, revealing how playful teaching and learning foster creative thinking, problem-solving, independence, and perseverance. It demonstrates how 'intellectually playful instruction might be a promising way to infuse high school classrooms with opportunities that support both rigor and pleasure' (Fine 2014: 8), promoting intrinsic goals with the associated positive implications for students' mental health and wellbeing.

Box 5.4 Too old to play? Acknowledging the importance of playful thinking in the high school

Alistair Pugh

Older children love to play. They might turn their noses up at the thought of chasing each other around the playground, or climbing trees, or bouncing balls – but they still play because they're still curious (Figure 5.1). But whereas younger children often like to test their physical limits, older children tend to spend more time 'in their heads'. They test their mental limits: experimenting with emotions and relationships; dabbling with ideals and questioning beliefs. Teenagers are especially playful when it comes to speech. Many of the new words that come into the language every year are coined by young people. It's creative – and subversive. When young people play with language, they demonstrate their sophisticated understanding of common 'rules', ideas, and sounds and their ability to apply them in innovative new ways. Playful thinkers – think of Einstein or Mozart – are more likely to be the sort of people who bend or break the 'rules' by asking: 'what would happen if?' They have the confidence to try out new ideas. It's no accident that physicists and mathematicians tend to make their biggest breakthroughs before they reach the age of 30.

Unfortunately, while teenagers have a natural gift for creative thinking, conventional educational tasks often suppress it. The culture of getting 'the right answer' and of 'teaching to the test' in a high-stakes system where exam results are the gold standard measure of 'progress' means that, whereas the instinct of most teenagers is to experiment with new thinking, their experimentation is discredited because the process of 'learning by mistakes' goes unrecognized. This lowers confidence and generates anxiety, discouraging engagement. But it doesn't have to be like that.

In my work as a geography teacher at Edinburgh Steiner School, I am fortunate to be able to teach some courses (called Main Lessons) purely to expand the horizons of the learners, rather than to prepare the students for examination. World Geography is one of the Main Lessons I teach to Class 12 (ages 17–18). In this Main Lesson – taught over the course of four weeks, for an hour and twenty minutes every day – we explore big, complex ideas (terrorism; globalization; urban poverty; gender) and there are no 'right' answers. I want my pupils to have the confidence to play around with different ideas and not to be discouraged when their proposed 'solution' to a global issue doesn't quite stand up to the rigorous questioning of their classmates. This is easier because there's no textbook and no test.

The World Geography Main lesson is often taught in the Autumn term, during the weeks of Advent, so I created a short rhythmic activity known as the World Geography Advent Calendar, using a prop made out of cardboard and decorated with crudely rendered drawings of iconic landmarks and natural wonders. To account for weekends, and because the term ends a few days before Christmas, students would take turns to open two doors at the start of every lesson. Behind each door they would find a mini map of a country and, as its name was announced, they would race to be the first to identify and shout out its capital city. There were small prizes for the winners, and I would then tell them something interesting about each country and try to answer any questions.

The students were told at the outset that the countries behind the doors of the calendar were not randomly selected: there was a pattern. This was a game and, if they wanted to play (which most of them did), they must take a careful note of all the countries and the order in which they were revealed. I told them that behind door number 24, to be opened on the last day of term, there was the name of a famous town. The first person to figure out the pattern, crack the 'code', and correctly guess the name of the town would get a prize. The 'pattern' was difficult to spot early on; jumping from Vanuatu, to Uruguay, to Lesotho, but eventually the pupils would notice that the countries were clustered around the Mediterranean, in a rough spiral. The town behind door number 24 was Bethlehem.

The main purpose of this activity is to give learners an opportunity to experiment with ideas in a free and fun way. Over the years, I have been presented with some impressive 'theories' regarding the pattern of the countries: I have been confidently informed that anagrams of the countries' names point to 'Toronto', or that a mathematical solution involving the averages of distances between second cities suggests 'Lagos'. It didn't matter that these theories were way off the mark: students were learning by applying knowledge and testing ideas in a risk-free activity. When pupils play in this way, using trial and error, they are engaged in a heuristic learning process in which they are free to ask the crucial question: 'what would happen if . . .?'

Teachers are given a golden opportunity to harness the power of play to make learning fun. But it requires that our school systems let young people try and fail by recognizing and rewarding the learning process itself. For as long as failure remains a thing to be ashamed of, young people won't stop playing – they'll simply play somewhere else.

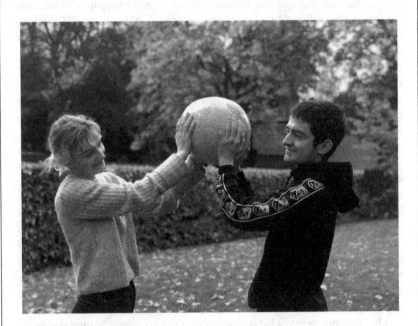

Figure 5.1 Older children still love to play

Source: Photograph by Sarah Miller.

Socialization in the digital playground

Play in adolescence is predominantly social, and it meets the young person's need to find their place in the group and ultimately in the world. Through play, teenagers continue to develop and refine the social skills involved in communication, such as negotiation, cooperation, and sharing, along with coping skills such as perseverance and self-regulation. However, it has always been the case that 'the search for identity, experience and meaning leads to play behaviours that can sometimes be at odds with adults expectations' (Robinson 2014: 6).

The rapid rise in the use of mobile digital technology over the past decade means that most social play in adolescence now takes place in cyberspace, leading to concerns that teens are missing out on opportunities to develop key social and relationship skills and are placing themselves at risk of serious mental harm (Twenge 2017). While there are clear contraindications for the use of digital media in childhood (as discussed in Chapter 4), the picture for adolescents is more nebulous.

There is a robust body of evidence that mobile phone use disrupts the quality and quantity of sleep in adolescence (Fuller et al. 2017), with negative implications for young people's physical and mental health. There is also widespread concern about the impact of cyberbullying on youth mental health (Athanasiou et al. 2018). Research shows an overlap between online and offline bullying (Kowalski et al. 2014), but the anonymity and unlimited access offered by the internet can exacerbate the problem of aggressive victimization. Viner et al. (2019) examined the association between the frequency of social media use and mental health and wellbeing in adolescence. They found that the negative impact of frequent social media use is primarily attributable to the displacement of sleep and physical activity and to exposure to cyberbullying.

Twenge and Campbell (2019) report that teens who spend a lot of time on social media engage in fewer person-to-person interactions and, as a result, feel more lonely and less able to cope with stress and anxiety. This is similar to Greenfield's (2014: 265) argument that 'social networking sites could worsen communication skills and reduce interpersonal empathy'. Even more alarmingly, neuroscientist, Frances Jensen (2015) regards the use of smartphones, and engagement with social media, as a form of addiction to which teenage brains are particularly vulnerable. A study by Crone and Konijn (2018) explains that the neural systems associated with the use of digital social media remain 'underdeveloped and undergoing significant changes during adolescence' and 'may make them specifically reactive to emotion-arousing media', supporting the view that parents and elders continue to have a vital role in adolescence for setting boundaries and finding opportunities to build resilience.

However, research also shows that, while time spent online commonly displaces real-time contact with family and friends, regular virtual communication can also strengthen the quality of existing relationships (Davis 2012). Bryant et al. (2006) found that there was considerable overlap between online and offline friendships, and an analysis of virtual exchanges by Underwood et al.

(2015) showed that most online communication in adolescence involves positive (or neutral) interactions between friends. There is a view that socializing and playing online is less meaningful than offline play and socializing, but Taylor (2020) makes the case that our online experiences have become so interwoven with our everyday lives – at personal, educational, professional, and societal levels – that the overlap has become increasingly blurred.

For teenage boys especially, online interactions (in particular those related to gaming) can facilitate social communication that they might find hard in real life. Ben (aged 12) explains: 'It is often easier to talk with people whilst you are doing something you both enjoy, and it stops there from having to be constant chat to make it not seem awkward'. He adds that when engaged with a friend in an online game, they 'chat about the game – and life'. With the wisdom of youth, Ben recognizes that 'being with each other is better for you' but adds that meeting up with friends online 'means it can happen more often . . . and you feel like you are with them, instead of having to make an effort to meet somewhere every day'.

Bandura (1997) suggests that cognition and behavior are functions of both human agency and the social context (DiBenedetto and Bembenutty 2013). Our personal thoughts and feelings influence the way we behave in relation to the social environment, and our behavior refines the way we think and feel about ourselves and our place in the world. When teens begin to move away from the familiar circle of home and school, they need to adapt their behavior to a whole new set of social mores and variable contexts. As a valuable source of behavioral feedback, play offers young people a means of finding and validating their place in the wider community. In the next case-story, Debbie Tonkin reflects on how being part of a play community during her university years reinforced her self-belief and self-regulatory behaviors.

Box 5.5 Gathering the magic: finding fun and companionship through role-play and gaming

Debbie Tonkin

While at University, I was introduced to a game called *Magic: The Gathering* (MTG). MTG is a trading card game for ages 13 and up, which involves building a deck of 60 cards, to attack with creature cards and deal damage with spells to reduce your opponent's life total from 20 to 0 (there are other ways to win and other formats of the game, but this is the general aim in its most simplistic form). I was hooked from the first time I played, and my free time was soon consumed with playing tabletop *Magic*, with the tips earned from my waitressing job spent on buying booster packs of cards.

As I became better at the game, I started to attend local gaming store events called 'pre-releases', where players are given early access to new sets of cards one week before the official release, and *Friday Night Magic* (FNM), a casual weekly event. Attending these events introduced me to a wide range of *Magic* players in the local community. I have played against Juniors, non-English-speaking opponents, and a cross section of people with disabilities, including visual impairment. The community around the game is what made it for me. As someone who has never really felt like I 'fitted in' to society, it was a new experience to be able to come together with people of different ages, cultures, and backgrounds and to feel as if I belonged. It didn't matter where I went – Reading where I went to university, Cheltenham where my best friend lived, or London where my family live – the game is played with the same rules and regulations, and there are fantastic communities built around playing it.

After playing the game for two years, I decided to try out a new gaming store which had opened close to my home. A small group of us began to attend competitions at the weekends, which led to us searching for more competitive events around the south of the country. We would gather at 6 a.m. and drive an hour or so away to participate at different gaming stores, where we got to know the local store owners and other competitors. This escalated to attending 2,500+ player events called Grand Prix. Without playing *Magic: The Gathering*, I would never have traveled to Warsaw, Madrid, or Utrecht with a group of friends.

As someone with a tendency to love organization, filing, and collecting, the range of accessories to the game, including binders, boxes, and card sleeves, all appealed to me as much as the playing. Every town my mum and I visited for weekends away or shopping trips involved a mission to find the local MTG retailer to buy and open some booster packs.

The local gaming store community is one reliant on play, and its customer base, myself included, are thankful for the time, effort, and safe space provided by the owners and tournament organizers. *Magic: The Gathering* is but one of a huge number of games with a strong community built around play.

It may come across that I spent my student years gaming, however I did come away with an Upper Second-Class degree in History and a Masters in Medieval Studies! Knowing that I had Magic events to look forward to in my free time, allowed me to really focus on my studies the rest of the time.

There is a case to be made that engaging in social play and interaction through a digital medium can help to build and develop the social skills which some young people may struggle with in the real world. Games specifically targeted at children and teens with social–behavioral problems, such as *Adventures Aboard the S.S. GRIN* (3C Institute n.d.a), have demonstrated improvements in 'social literacy, social anxiety, bullying victimization, social satisfaction, psychosocial stress, and behavioral and emotional strength'. Other games and media plat-forms, such as *My Kidney Guru* (3C Institute n.d.b), which are aimed at ado-lescents with specific health conditions, deploy recognizably playful learning strategies to address health literacy and treatment compliance issues.

However, even mainstream video games contain many of the archetypal fea-tures of traditional play with which young people identify, and observation and analysis of their digital play choices and behaviors can offer valuable insight into their emotional disposition. This is illustrated in the following case-story by Laura Walsh, who describes how a shared gaming experience became a power-ful means of communication for a young person in hospital. The game came to represent a metaphor for the adolescent struggle for identity and autonomy, revealing deep feelings that evaded verbal expression.

Box 5.6 Pixelated play: it's all in the game

Laura Walsh

Technology. It can strike fear into the heart of the play purist and create spine-tingling shivers in those who mourn the depletion of the type of play they believe to be nourishing for children and young people. The modern world can seem to be lacking in opportunities to connect in the physical realm: freedom to roam, fresh air, or simple pleasures. But the lure of 'simpler times' can sometimes cloud the judgment of our adult minds as we fail to recognize the meaning in the play that is happening right in front of our eyes.

Lawrence, 14-year-old, has been admitted to hospital countless times and become what is known as a 'long termer'. On one occasion he is unaccompanied and, although his parents visit as often as they can, he spends a lot of time alone. He loves to play video games and when a console is available to him, he remains glued to it. Lawrence has a good relationship with the Playworker on his ward and, although gaming is not really her thing, she sometimes joins him for a game of Super Mario, usually taking the parts of the more devious characters and accepting easy defeat. When play becomes more multilayered, she performs less badly in the game, creating a more surprising route toward identifying with notions of success and failure. More than 'just a game' this play opens up potential ways of exploring identity, strategy, competitiveness, and ego bruising/soothing.

In the course of these episodes of parallel play, conversation occasion-ally turns to Lawrence's feelings and, like the richness that can transpire through conversation on a long car journey, there are profound moments of emotional reveal. While immersed in the game world, playing as individuals but together, they find a way to traverse the awkward space between them. Filling that space with simple actions and busy hands, maneuvering vehicles and avatars along ravines and through caverns, they reach something deeper, a kind of togetherness, without fanfare or ceremony. A way to connect to self and other.

During one play session the Playworker was surprised to find Lawrence come across as snappy and rude as he pushed aside her suggested activity for the day, barked that he wanted to finish his game on his own, and asked for the window blinds to stay closed for the rest of the day. Taken aback by his outburst, she brought her feeling of rejection to a reflective practice session and described how she had responded, what she felt, and the outcome of the interaction. Lawrence's out-of-character behavior could have been simply dismissed as typical of a game-obsessed teen but, on deeper reflection, it seemed that he wanted to share the important message that he felt boundary-less and unsafe or uncared for. Much more than 'just playing', the Playworker's relationship with Lawrence, built up through a shared play experience, allowed him to communicate his feelings of vulnerability and abandonment and opened our eyes to the value of the game.

For most adolescents, digital media devices have become a tool for engaging in routine exchanges with friends and for strengthening existing relationships, while much of their play often takes place in a virtual play space. However, this is still new territory which demands a balancing of the risks and benefits. The American Academy of Pediatrics (2020) recommends that parents help to prioritize sleep and physical activity, establish screen-free times and zones, and engage in digital content along with their teens. Dr Michael Rich of Harvard University (cited at Center for Humane Technology 2020) advocates the 'empty glass' exercise for parents to help their teens prioritize a healthy lifestyle:

> Thinking of their day as an empty glass, they should fill it with the essentials; enough sleep to grow and avoid getting sick, school, time to spend outdoors, play, socialize, do homework, and to sit down for one meal a day together as a family (perhaps the single most protective thing you can do to keep their bodies and minds healthy). Once these activities are totaled, remaining time can be used for other experiences that interest the child, such as the activity in question (Minecraft, Fortnite etc.).

The concept of digital flourishing is 'a mindful approach to digital technology usage that supports our thriving in different areas of life. This approach empowers us to take advantage of the benefits of technology while avoiding associated harms' (The Digital Wellness Collective 2020). The Digital Flourishing Wheel shown in Figure 5.2 illustrates the ways in which we can all enhance our wellbeing across six domains affected by our digital engagement, and each of these intersects with the play principles at the heart of this chapter.

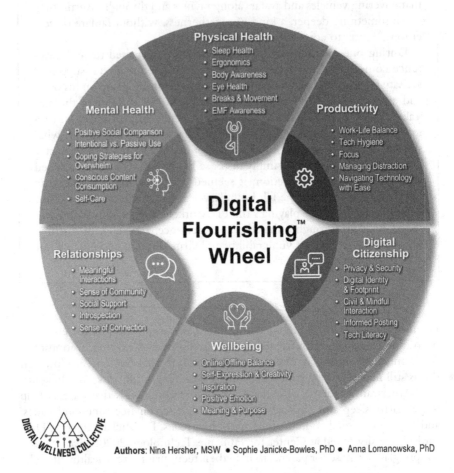

Figure 5.2 The Digital Flourishing Wheel (Digital Wellness Collective 2020)

Source: Reproduced by kind permission of the Digital Wellness Collective.

Young people growing up in the twenty-first century are bombarded with competing demands on their attention; learning to act with awareness and intention, rather than simply reacting to the buzz of external stimuli, helps teens to make wise, informed choices which will support their ability 'to focus, to delay gratification, to form identity, form meaningful relationships, and to maintain mental health' (Center for Humane Technology 2020).

Conclusion

Adolescence is the transitional stage between childhood and adulthood encompassing major biological development and the growth of social roles and relationships. During this period, adolescents require nurturing, secure environments that facilitate the growth of resilience and a positive sense of who they are, as well as a need to be valued for what they have to offer to their community and society as a whole. Parents continue to be a significant part of their child's life and playful endeavors provide a conduit for sharing experiences and communication at a time when boundaries are tested, and logical thought processes are still being developed. Adolescence, rich with creativity and innovation, is the ideal time for exploration through play, which supports the drive for self-discovery and the development of personal identity.

References

3C Institute (n.d.a) *Adventures Aboard the S.S. GRIN*. Online. HTTP: <www.3cisd.com/online-social-skills-game-for-children> (accessed 12 October 2020).

3C Institute (n.d.b) *Living with CKD: An E-Learning Platform for Adolescents with CKD about the Disease and Its Management*. Online. HTTP: <www.3cisd.com/portfolio/living-with-ckd-an-e-learning-platform-for-adolescents-with-ckd-about-the-disease-and-its-management/> (accessed 12 October 2020).

Ackerman, D. (1999) *Deep Play*. New York: Vintage Books.

Alimujiang, A., Wiensch, A., Boss, J., Fleischer, N., Mondul, A., McLean, K., Mukherjee, B. and Leigh Pearce, C. (2019) Association between life purpose and mortality among US adults older than 50 years. *JAMA Network Open*, 2 (5): e194270. doi:10.1001/jamanetworkopen.2019.4270.

American Academy of Pediatrics (2020) *American Academy of Pediatrics Announces New Recommendations for Children's Media Use*. Online. HTTP: <https://services.aap.org/en/news-room/news-releases/aap/2016/aap-announces-new-recommendations-for-media-use/> (accessed 12 October 2020).

Arain, M., Haque, M., Johal, L., Mathur, P., Nel, W., Rais, A., Sandhu, R. and Sharma, S. (2013) Maturation of the adolescent brain. *Neuropsychiatric Disease and Treatment*, 9: 449–461. doi.org/10.2147/NDT.S39776.

Athanasiou, K., Melegkovits, E., Andrie, E. K., Charalampos, M., Chara, K., Richardson, C., Greydanus, D., Tsolia, M. and Tsitsika, A. (2018) Cross-national aspects of cyberbullying victimization among 14–17-year-old adolescents across seven European countries. *BMC Public Health*, 18: 800. Online. HTTP: <https://bmcpublichealth.biomedcentral.com/articles/10.1186/s12889-018-5682-4> (accessed 10 October 2020).

Aubrun, A. and Grady, J. (2000) *Reframing Youth: Models, Metaphors, Messages*. Online. HTTP: https://frameworksinstitute.org/assets/files/PDF/youth_reframing.pdf (accessed 24 February 2020).

Bandura, A. (1997) *Self-Efficacy: The Exercise of Control*. New York: Freeman.

Benson, P. L. (2008) *Sparks: How Parents Can Help Ignite the Hidden Strengths of Teenagers*. San Francisco, CA: Jossey-Bass.

Biddulph, S. (2013) *Steve Biddulph's Raising Girls*. Sydney: Finch.

Biddulph, S. (2015) *Raising Boys: Why Boys Are Different – and How to Help Them Become Happy and Well-Balanced Men*. London: Thorsons.

Biddulph, S. (2017) *10 Things Girls Need Most: To Grow Up Strong and Free*. London: Harper Thorsons.

Boykin McElhaney, K., Allen, J. P., Stephenson, J. C. and Hare, A. L. (2009) Attachment and autonomy during adolescence. In: Lerner, R. M. and Steinberg, L. (Eds.), *Handbook of Adolescent Psychology*. New Jersey: Wiley.

Breuner, C. C. and Levine, D. A. (2017) AAP Committee on adolescence: Adolescent and young adult tattooing, piercing, and scarification. *Pediatrics*, 140 (4): e20171962.

Bryant, J. A., Sanders-Jackson, A. and Smallwood, A. M. K. (2006) IMing, text messaging, and adolescent social networks. *Journal of Computer-Mediated Communication*, 11 (2): 577–592.

Carter, R. (2018) *The Brain in Minutes: 200 Key Ideas of Neuroscience Explained in an Instant*. London: Quercus.

Center for Humane Technology (2020) *Digital Well-Being Guidelines for Parents during the COVID-19 Pandemic*. Online. HTTP: <www.humanetech.com/digital-wellbeing-covid> (accessed 21 November 2020).

Child Trends (2018) *Violent Crime Victimization*. Online. HTTP: <www.childtrends.org/indicators/violent-crime-victimization> (accessed 24 February 2020).

Conklin, H. G. (2015) *Playtime Isn't Just for Preschoolers: Teenagers Need It, Too*. Online. HTTP: <https://time.com/3726098/learning-through-play-teenagers-education/> (accessed 23 February 2020).

Crone, E. A. and Konijn, E. A. (2018) Media use and brain development during adolescence. *Nature Communications*, 9: 588. doi:10.1038/s41467-018-03126-x.

Damon, W., Menon, J. and Bronk, K. C. (2003) The development of purpose during adolescence. *Applied Developmental Science*, 7 (3): 119–128.

Davis, K. (2012) Friendship 2.0: Adolescents' experiences of belonging and self-disclosure online. *Journal of Adolescence*, 35 (6): 1527–1536.

De Koven, B. (2013) *The Well-Played Game: A Player's Philosophy*. Cambridge, MA: MIT Press.

De Koven, B. (2017) Of playfulness and play: We must play because it is as necessary to us as breathing: We are born players. *Psychology Today*. Online. HTTP: <www.psychologytoday.com/gb/blog/having-fun/201704/playfulness-and-play> (accessed 26 August 2020).

DiBenedetto, M. K. and Bembenutty, H. (2013) Within the pipeline: Self-regulated learning, self-efficacy, and socialization among college students in science courses. *Journal of Psychology and Education: Learning and Individual Differences*, 23: 218–224.

The Digital Wellness Collective (2020) *What Is Digital Wellness?* Online. HTTP: <https://digitalwellnesscollective.com/digitalwellness> (accessed 10 October 2020).

Douglas, L. (2020a) *The Poet Helping Young People of Colour Explore Their Identity through Verse*. Online. HTTP: <www.positive.news/lifestyle/arts/poetry-can-articulate-our-complexities-theresa-lola-on-language-and-identity/?utm_source=Positive+News&utm_campaign=4793dd3f80-EMAIL_CAMPAIGN_2020_10_09_10_43&utm_medium=email&utm_term=0_3a293415a0-4793dd3f80-341336060> (accessed 13 October 2020).

Douglas, L. (2020b) *The Artist Helping Black Teenage Boys Feel Seen, Heard and Inspired*. Online. HTTP: <www.positive.news/lifestyle/the-artist-helping-young-black-boys-feel-seen-heard-and-inspired/?utm_source=Positive+News&utm_campaign=4793dd3f80-EMAIL_CAMPAIGN_2020_10_09_10_43&utm_medium=email&utm_term=0_3a293415a0-4793dd3f80-341336060> (accessed 13 October 2020).

Fine, S. M. (2014) 'A slow revolution': Toward a theory of intellectual playfulness in high school classrooms. *Harvard Educational Review*, 84 (1): 1–23.

Fuller, C., Lehman, E., Hicks, S. and Novick, M. B. (2017) Bedtime use of technology and associated sleep problems in children. *Global Pediatric Health*. Online. HTTP: <https://doi.org/10.1177/2333794X17736972> (accessed 10 October 2020).

Galinsky, E. (1999) *Ask the Children: What America's Children Really Think about Working Parents*. New York: William Morrow and Co.

Gray, P. (2011) The decline of play and the rise of psychopathology in children and adolescents. *American Journal of Play*, 3 (4): 443–463.

Greenfield, S. (2014) *Mind Change: How Digital Technologies Are Leaving Their Mark on Our Brains*. London: Rider.

Happiness Research Institute (2020) Online. HTTP: <www.happinessresearchinstitute.com/> (accessed 13 October 2020).

Hooker, S. A., Masters, K. S. and Park, C. L. (2018) A meaningful life is a healthy life: A conceptual model linking meaning and meaning salience to health. *Review of General Psychology*, 22 (1): 11–24.

Jager, J., Yuen, C. X., Putnick, D. L., Hendricks, C. and Bornsteinn, M. H. (2015) Adolescent peer relationships, separation and detachment from parents, and internalizing and externalizing behaviors: Linkages and interactions. *Journal of Early Adolescence*, 35: 511–537.

Jensen, F. E. (2015) *The Teenage Brain: A Neuroscientist's Survival Guide to Raising Adolescent*. London: Harper Collins.

Jewell, J. D., Axelrod, M. I., Prinstein, M. J. and Hupp, S. (2018) *Great Myths of Adolescence*. Hoboken, NJ: Wiley-Blackwell.

Johnston, L. D., O'Malley, P. M., Meich, R. A., Bachman, J. G. and Schulenberg, J. E. (2016) *Monitoring the Future National Survey Results on Drug Use, 1975–2016: Overview, Key Findings on Adolescent Drug Use*. Ann Arbor, MI: Institute for Social Research, The University of Michigan.

Kane, P. (n.d.) *What Is 'The Play Ethic'?* Online. HTTP: <www.theplayethic.com/what-is-the-play-ethic.html> (accessed 13 October 2020).

Kasser, T. (2002) *The High Price of Materialism*. Cambridge, MA: MIT Press.

Kowalski, R. M., Giumetti, G. W., Schroeder, A. N. and Lattanner, M. R. (2014) Bullying in the digital age: A critical review and meta-analysis of cyberbullying research among youth. *Psychological Bulletin*. doi:10.1037/a0035618.

Kubik, J., Docherty, M. and Boxer, P. (2019) The impact of childhood maltreatment on adolescent gang involvement. *Childhood Abuse and Neglect*, 96: 10496.

Make Time 2 Play (2020) *Adolescents: 13–19 Years*. Online. HTTP: <www.maketime2play.co.uk/fun-forever/adolescents/> (accessed 5 October 2020).

Mental Health Foundation (2020) *Mental Health Statistics: Children and Young People*. Online. HTTP: <www.mentalhealth.org.uk/statistics/mental-health-statistics-children-and-young-people> (accessed 24 February 2020).

National Scientific Council on the Developing Child (2015) *Supportive Relationships and Active Skill-Building Strengthen the Foundations of Resilience*. Working Paper No. 13. Online. HTTP: <https://46y5eh11fhgw3ve3ytpwxt9r-wpengine.netdna-ssl.com/wp-content/uploads/2015/05/The-Science-of-Resilience2.pdf> (accessed 4 September 2020).

Office for National Statistics (2013) *Drinking, in General Lifestyle Survey, 2011*. Online. HTTP: <www.ons.gov.uk/peoplepopulationandcommunity/personalandhouseholdfinances/incomeandwealth/compendium/generallifestylesurvey/2013-03-07> (accessed 20 November 2020).

Paediatric Society of New Zealand (2020) *Adolescent Brain Development*. Online. HTTP: <www.kidshealth.org.nz/adolescent-brain-development> (accessed 22 June 2020).

Perry, P. (2020) *The Book You Wish Your Parents Had Read (and Your Children Will Be Glad That You Did)*. New York: Pamela Dorman Books.

Project Trust (2020) *Where Will You Go?* Online. HTTP: <https://projecttrust.org.uk/> (accessed 20 November 2020).

Robinson, M. (2014) *Grounds for Learning: 11–18 Secondary School Play: The Research behind Play in Schools*. Online. HTTP: <www.londonplay.org.uk/resources/0000/1737/The_value_of_play_in_11-18_secondary_schools_Jan_2015.pdf> (accessed 9 October 2020).

Schwartz, S. E., Lowe, S. R. and Rhodes, J. E. (2012) Mentoring relationships and adolescent self-esteem. *Prevention Research*, 19 (2): 17–20.

Science Direct (2020) *Synaptogenesis*. Online. HTTP: <www.sciencedirect.com/topics/neuroscience/synaptogenesis> (accessed 23 June 2020).

Seligman, M. (2011) *Authentic Happiness*. Online. HTTP: <www.authentichappiness.sas.upenn.edu/learn/wellbeing> (accessed 27 February 2020).

Shaw, S. K. and Dallos, R. (2005) Attachment and adolescent depression: The impact of early attachment experiences. *Attachment and Human Development*, 7 (4): 409–424.

Siegel, D. (2014) Dopamine and teenage logic. *The Atlantic*. Online. HTTP: <www.theatlantic.com/health/archive/2014/01/dopamine-and-teenage-logic/282895/> (accessed 3 September 2020).

Sissay, L. (2019) *My Name Is Why*. Edinburgh: Canongate.

Speck, D. (2018) 'He Opened Up the World to Me': Ian Wright on Primary Teacher. Online. HTTP: <www.tes.com/news/he-opened-world-me-ian-wright-primary-teacher> (accessed 28 February 2020).

Steinberg, L. (2014) *Age of Opportunity: Lessons from the New Science of Adolescence*. Boston: Houghton Mifflin Harcourt.

Suttie, J. (2016) *What Adolescents Really Need from Parents*. Online. HTTP: <https://greatergood.berkeley.edu/article/item/what_adolescents_really_need_from_parents> (accessed 17 May 2020).

Taylor, T. L. (2020) The rise of massive multiplayer online games, esports, and game live streaming. *American Journal of Play*, 12 (2): 107–116.

Twenge, J. M. (2017) *Have Smartphones Destroyed a Generation?* Online. HTTP: <www.theatlantic.com/magazine/archive/2017/09/has-the-smartphone-destroyed-a-generation/534198/> (accessed 10 October 2020).

Twenge, J. M. and Campbell, W. K. (2019) Digital media use is linked to lower psychological well-being: Evidence from three datasets. *Psychiatric Quarterly*, 90: 311–331.

Underwood, M. K., Ehrenreich, S. E., More, D., Solis, J. S. and Brinkley, D. Y. (2015) The BlackBerry Project: The hidden world of adolescents' text messaging and relations with internalizing symptoms. *Journal of Research on Adolescence*, 25 (1): 101–117. doi:10.1111/jora.12101.

universalsoulartist (2019) *S.M.I.L.E-ing Boys Project*. Online. HTTP: <http://universoulartist.com/smiling-boys-project/> (accessed 13 October 2020).

Viner, R. M., Greesh, A., Stiglic, N., Hudson, L. D., Goddings, A.-L., Ward, J. L. and Nicholls, D. E. (2019) Roles of cyberbullying, sleep, and physical activity in mediating the effects of social media use on mental health and wellbeing among young people in England: A secondary analysis of longitudinal data. *The Lancet, Child and Adolescent Health*, 3 (10): 685–696.

Whitaker, J. (2019) Finding playfulness in the everyday: An antidote to the 'saturation' of modern family life. In: Tonkin, A. and Whitaker, J. (Eds.), *Play and Playfulness for Public Health and Wellbeing*. Oxon: Routledge: 92–103.

6   Early adulthood

The brain is a highly complex, integrated organ that coordinates multiple functions using brain architecture which results from the interaction of our genes and the environment at every stage of the life course (Center on the Developing Child 2020). After the rapid and dynamic changes associated with adolescence, Lawton (2009) describes how we enter the 'fourth age of the brain' at around 22 years of age. This is the age at which the brain is deemed to reach adulthood, remaining at the peak of its powers for just five years (*ibid.*). At 25 years of age, the brain is at its heaviest, weighing in at around 1.3 kg, and the ability to store, cross-reference, and recall information reaches an optimal level (Coast 2016). The prefrontal cortex known as the 'seat of executive decision making' reaches maturation, completing the remodeling of the brain. The young adult is now able to control their impulses, to prioritize, to plan, and to organize their life such that they can achieve their goals (Cummins 2017). But Lawton (2009) cautions us to 'enjoy it while it lasts [because] from there it's downhill all the way', and he goes on to outline the long, slow decline in brain functionality which will follow throughout the adult years.

Age-associated, non-pathological, cognitive decline is part of our human experience and, as with all changes in functionality, the extent of change differs between individuals (Deary et al. 2009). Most research into cognitive functionality seems to focus on the negative effects of brain deterioration over time. After the age of 27 years, this is manifest in a rapid decline in episodic memory, planning, and task coordination; a slowing down in processing speed; and reduced capacity to store information (Lawton 2009). This deterioration is not uniform across all areas of the brain and different abilities will decline at varying rates (*ibid.*). However, Dinishak (2016) remarks that this *deficit view* of brain development 'diminishes people's life chances and even their humanity' and that 'On this line of criticism, challenging deficit thinking is seen as a moral imperative'. Reframing developmental change in a positive light allows us to notice and to appreciate different aspects of the brain's potential at each life stage and 'what happens when we appreciate some-thing or [some-] one . . . it gets better. More precious. More fun' (De Koven 2014: 23).

In her critique of the deficit model of individual differences, Dinishak (2016) uses the example of autism to discuss how the labeling arising from a deficit perspective both impacts the personal and social identities of individuals and impedes the progress of professional understanding. Focusing on the decrease, loss, or absence of certain capacities over time fails to appreciate the creative potential of alternative forms of functioning (Sass 2001) and denies opportunities for the creative development of professional practice.

Wilson (2017: 38) suggests that 'reaching towards creative practices involves an exploration of what we find stimulating and satisfying in the jobs that we do'. He identifies three interrelated dimensions to the potential for creative development: knowledge, style, and generous spirit. In the following case-story, experienced play specialist, Jenny Oliver, takes the risk of applying her knowledge and skills with 'generosity of spirit' in a novel context – by introducing therapeutic play into an adult setting – accepting the associated 'uncertainty in the belief that such a step will bring with it a degree of hope and new possibility' (Wilson 2017: p. 47).

Box 6.1 Building a tower of explanation: play as a healthcare intervention for adults with learning disabilities

Jenny Oliver

A hospital admission is a daunting prospect for most people, but for those with learning disabilities or autism it can be overwhelming. The unfamiliar hospital environment and sensory overload can be a source of extreme stress and anxiety, and communication challenges may inhibit effective interaction between the patient and healthcare team. As a Health Play Specialist, I have worked with many children with a learning disability or autism, using therapeutic play to facilitate a hospital stay or treatment procedure, and I have often worried how these patients fare when transferred to the care of adult services, when play is taken off the care plan. When I was invited to work with Harvey, I had a chance to explore whether there might also be a role for the Health Play Specialist in adult healthcare.

Harvey is a 25-year-old man with a diagnosis of moderate learning difficulties and autism. He lives at home with his mother and an older sister and relies on their interpretation of his nonverbal behavior to communicate his needs and wishes, as well as using Makaton signing. Harvey attends a day center where he enjoys music, art, and sensory activities, especially dancing and singing along to his favorite tunes.

I met Harvey for the first time on the day of his surgery and found him calm and content, listening to music in the company of his mother and sibling. In conversation with the family, we agreed that the most helpful thing for Harvey would be to explain what was going to happen by breaking the process down into its component steps. This led to the building of 'a tower of explanation' constructed from colored blocks, each of which represented a different stage in Harvey's hospital journey (Figure 6.1). Each element of the surgical process was depicted using different colored symbols and short explanatory statements and, as each stage was completed, Harvey removed a block from the tower. This graphic representation of the passage of time allowed Harvey to process

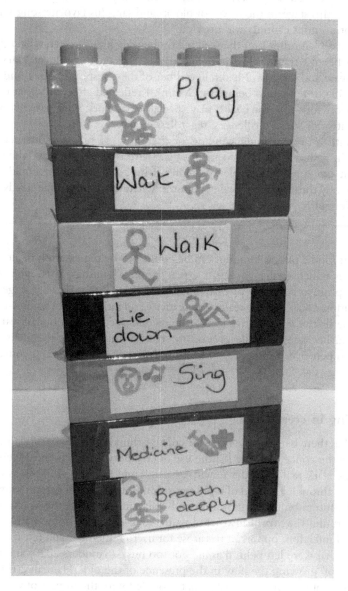

Figure 6.1 Harvey's 'tower of explanation'

Source: Photograph by Jenny Oliver.

essential information in a gradual and manageable way and to monitor his own progress throughout the day.

While Harvey waited for his allocated theatre slot, we played video games, sang familiar songs, and read books, establishing a therapeutic rapport as cooperative playmates. In the anesthetic room, Harvey indicated that he wanted me to stay close. Speaking softly and calmly, I reminded him of this stage in the tower of blocks and sang his favorite song while an intravenous cannula was inserted.

Harvey's mother later thanked me for helping him through what might have been a traumatic experience. By taking on the role of Harvey's advocate and support, I had relieved her of these responsibilities, and she was able to relax into being just 'Mum'. I reflected afterwards that there is an obvious role for health play specialists to work with patients with cognitive or social challenges, regardless of age.

With a greater understanding of the value of play for our general health, it should not be surprising that there is a role for play when we are at our most vulnerable. Wouldn't it be good if *everyone* could play their way through a hospital encounter, whatever their unique needs and challenges?

A deficit model of development can be countered by the creation of alternative narratives which challenge negative perceptions (Dinishak 2016) and support a more positive portrayal of early adulthood and all that this life stage has to offer – most notably in the realms of creativity and innovation. The mid-twenties mark the first of two creative peaks (the second occurring in our fifties), when the brain becomes a fertile ground for radical innovation dependent on the ability to perceive, appreciate, and act on deviations from existing conventions (Weinberg et al. 2019).

Growing in creativity

Never has there been a time riper for creative thinking because 'fundamental to living in the conceptual age [is] the use of creativity' (Warner and Myers 2009: 29). The stark reality of the Covid-19 pandemic of 2020 reminds us that we are living through a period of rapid transition from an era of certain knowledge toward a future built on innovation and collaboration (Pink 2007). As governments around the world instructed us to 'lock-down' at home to reduce the spread of infection, opportunities arose for us 'to remember and relearn ways of creating that were left behind as life got too busy' (Saunders 2020) and to look for ways of 'growing the new in the presence of the old' (Hannah 2014: 131).

A constantly changing social climate coupled with the impact of years of fiscal austerity on the public sector mean that those of us working in education, health and social care have to adopt greater flexibility in the application of our theoretical approaches, as we attempt to find new ways of connecting with our colleagues, the users of our services – and with our own needs as practitioners. Creative practice, in the context of health and social care, recognizes value in the different skills and capacities of each player in an interaction and 'a belief in the creative power of each person' (Wilson 2017: 51). But an individual's capacity for creativity is not just determined psychologically: it also depends on their place in the wider social system, their personal history (including play history), and the opportunities and resources available to them. A systems model of creativity recognizes that it is these factors in the social and cultural environment which both enable and constrain creative practice (Csikszentmihalyi 1999).

Creativity can be defined as 'the capacity to produce ideas that are both original and adaptive' (Simonton 2001) and is clearly a quality which is not only necessary for physical and social survival in the modern world, but which 'can also result in major contributions to human civilization' (*ibid.*). Csikszentmihalyi (2013: 28) speaks of creativity as having the power to 'transform an existing domain into a new one' – by offering alternative perspectives and novel responses to questions and problems. Piaget (cited in Elkind 2007: 3) encapsulated the overlap between creativity and play in the quote: 'Play is the answer to the question, "How does anything new come about?"'.

Many studies have demonstrated that play, and having a playful attitude, contributes to the discovery of new, useful ideas (Brown 2008a, 2008b). The relationship between play and creativity hinges on the concept of divergent thinking – the capacity to generate multiple and varied responses to a set of stimuli (e.g., Russ and Kaugars 2010). We can recognize divergent thinking in the way children play with loose parts:

> A stick, for example, may become a fishing rod near real or imaginary water, a spurtle in a mud kitchen, a tool to nudge a football that is stuck in a tree; it can be thrown, floated, snapped, pinged, bent, hidden, added to a pile, burnt, tied to something else, split, catapulted or discarded.
>
> (Inspiring Scotland 2016)

Play links with creativity because it arouses emotion, and it is the emotional response which stimulates 'the originality of the divergent thinking responses' (Russ and Kaugars 2010).

With the transition from adolescence to early adulthood and the associated demands of academic achievement, job success, and new responsibilities, we can become so focused on finding a single, correct response to life's challenges that we lose the capacity for spontaneous exploration, because of our fear of somehow 'getting it wrong'. Perry (2014: 108) describes the 'child's unselfconscious joy in creativity' which can be lost as we get older, and Christensen (2014) observes that 'without a play-like attitude, creative insights hide from us behind fear and uncertainty'. Children play more freely when they feel secure in a trusted environment (Brown 2008b), and adults too need to be able to trust that their playfulness is permitted, accepted, and valued (De Koven 2014). Huizinga (1955) used the concept of 'the magic circle' to describe the protected space within which play takes place; because this 'play space' (physical or metaphorical) exists both in the real world yet separate from it, it offers a freedom of possibility from which creative insights can emerge and whereby fear of failure can be replaced by a psychological state of wonder and curiosity (Christensen 2014).

The widespread acceptance of the World Health Organization's (2020) definition of health as being more than simply the absence of illness has spurred interest in the fundamentals of holistic approaches to creating and sustaining health. Making the link between play and health recognizes the centrality of creativity to this connection. A comprehensive review by the All Party Parliamentary Group [APPG] on Arts Health and Wellbeing (2017: 20) showed that creativity can

> stimulate imagination and reflection; encourage dialogue with the deeper self and enable expression; change perspectives; contribute to the construction of identity; provoke cathartic release; provide a place of safety and freedom from judgement; yield opportunities for guided conversations; increase control over life circumstances; inspire change and growth; engender a sense of belonging; prompt collective working; and promote healing.

Perhaps most significantly, the report acknowledges creativity as a means of empowerment in the relationship people have with their own health and with the providers of services.

Adults are more likely to engage in *playful interactions* as opposed to *episodes of play*, but when they do engage in episodic play, this tends to be more prescribed and structured: 'examples include games, roleplaying, escape rooms and murder mystery parties' (Neale 2020: 29). Games, together with storytelling and the visual arts, represent the playful enactment of human creativity and have been used for engaging and enhancing learning opportunities in adult education and training since the early nineteenth century (*ibid.*). In the following case-story, Alison describes how a playful approach to teaching encourages divergent thinking while making learning fun.

Box 6.2 A Teddy Murder Mystery

Alison Tonkin

The Teddy Murder Mystery has been used numerous times as a playful activity designed to boost collaborative problem-solving and decision-making in groups of adult learners across a range of ages and educational levels.

Originally designed for Cub Scouts (at the time boys aged 8–10½) as part of a 'Detectives' themed evening, the Teddy Murder Mystery requires the solving of clues in order to identify the killer of an unfortunate victim. The only adaptation to the original game for teaching purposes is the replacement of a young Scout leader in the role of victim with a teddy bear – for obvious reasons.

How to play

Groups of students are invited to visit a murder scene, in which a number of suspects have been strategically placed. Props include a knife covered with blood (tomato ketchup) planted on one of the suspects, a toy syringe, and footprints leading to an open window (Figure 6.2). Six clues are scattered around the murder scene which, when considered together, make it obvious who the murderer is. Before surveying the scene, each group is given an envelope containing a set of simple instructions, a single coded message, and packets of chocolate buttons which may be exchanged with the teacher for hints on how to crack the code. The code reads:

9.20.23.1.19.20.8.5.13.15.14.11.5.25
(answer at the end of the story for those who want to play)

After spending five minutes examining the murder scene, the groups then have another ten minutes to consider the evidence before giving feedback to everybody else, including the identity of the murderer and the rationale for their decision. Without being told whether they have guessed correctly, and after listening to the feedback from other groups, they are then allowed a further five minutes to reconsider their verdict and rationale.

It is always entertaining to watch adults engaged in animated conversation while playing this game: as they explore the murder scene, try to solve the clues, and discuss their hypotheses. Conspiracy theories abound, with bizarre and elaborate plots revealing great imagination and creativity – but a complete disregard for the evidence!

The supply of chocolate is always a source of much delight and makes for the difficult decision of whether to exchange it for help in solving the coded message (which is actually a red herring, specially included to distract participants from the identity of the real killer).

Perhaps, the best part of the activity is when everyone is giving feedback. Groups listen intently to each other as they present their verdicts and the rationale for their decisions, but there can be lively disagreements as they challenge each other's deductive skills. Giving participants an extra five minutes to reconsider their original decision leads many groups, who correctly identify the killer the first time around, to change their minds – much to their annoyance when the true identity of the murderer is finally revealed.

For such a simple activity, which has been replicated many times, it is perhaps surprising that not one adult group has ever solved the murder *and* provided an accurate rationale . . . although plenty of deep learning (creative development of skills that can be used in new situations) has occurred amidst the fun.

To crack the code – 1 = A, 2 = B, 3 = C, 4 = D, etc. Would you have traded your chocolate buttons?

- **Instructions**
- **Chocolate buttons**
- **Evidence record sheet**
- **Variety of suspects**
- **One murder victim**
- **Room to set up the**

murder scene

Figure 6.2 Overview of the Teddy Murder Mystery

Source: Photograph by Alison Tonkin.

Breathing spaces

Early adulthood is a prime time for acquiring and refining the reserves of mental capital necessary for emotional and social cognition throughout adult life (Foresight Mental Capital and Wellbeing Project 2008). Neale (2020: 31) proposes that 'the variety, novelty and engagement' of a playful approach to early adult life 'may lead to the adaptive retention of cognitive functioning in later life' as well as helping to alleviate anxiety and depression.

Playful and creative practice in early adulthood can be seen to offer 'a breathing space' amidst the whirl of daily activity; an opportunity to 'open possibilities for continued development and inspiration' (Wilson 2017: 37). The following case-stories illustrate how a playful approach to health and wellbeing can break through logjams in our thinking, feeling, and doing and thus disrupt unhelpful patterns and reenergize the drive for change. In the next case-story Layla Tree describes a personal experience of the transformative nature of 'play in practice' as an exercise of the will which fosters personal resilience.

Box 6.3 Rediscovering the arts in the digital world

Layla Tree

The constant exposure by young people to, what Bernard Stiegler (2010) defines as the 'psychotechnologies', social media, gaming, and excessive screen time, is resulting in a lack of opportunity for the will of the individual to be tested. If you lose in a video game you just start again, the parameters will all be the same. But nature does not contain these fixed parameters. By giving an individual the opportunity to work with natural material, it is also exposing them to the possibility of failure. The wood may not respond how they expect it to, the yarn may tangle, the clay crack. It is how the individual deals with and subsequently learns from the experience that has the potential to change and carry them forward.

It is more important than ever that they are given the opportunity through education to experience and become engaged in practical skills in order to build resilience in everyday life.

I experienced this myself when I had the opportunity to try green woodworking on a pole lathe for the first time. I was excited and felt quite confident that this was something I would be good at. I listened carefully as the tutor explained how to stand in front of the lathe and meet it straight on, how to angle the chisel and apply the correct amount of pressure to the material, and that when everything was working in harmony the sound to listen out for as the material engaged with the tool.

To the skilled practitioner this skill, of engaging the body in order to work with and not fight against the material, becomes embedded. This process of embodying skills is described by Peter Korn (2013: 55): 'Over time he learns to read his material through its response to hand and tool. . . . Interpreting what he hears, feels and sees, the craftsman does not have the luxury of ambiguity'.

As I began working on the pole lathe, I could immediately see and feel the chisel bouncing on the wood, leaving deep, unsightly gashes in the material, quite unlike the beautiful smooth surface that Richard, our tutor, had achieved. I pressed the chisel in harder, my body moving to a position at right angles to the lathe. I found myself reacting physically and emotionally to the resistance the material was offering: I was sweating, and tears were pricking my eyes. The same feelings aroused when encountering conflict or difficult life situations.

Mary Richards (1989: 33) eloquently describes this process: 'As human beings functioning as potters, we centre ourselves and our clay. And we all know how necessary it is to be on centre ourselves if we wish to bring our clay "into centre" and not merely to agitate or bully it'. This was the resistance I was meeting; I was forcing my will onto the material 'bullying it' (*ibid.*) rather than engaging my hands and body to feel and listen for the intrinsic properties of the wood.

A pause. A space in the journey. I stepped away from my lathe and waited. The physical and emotional manifestations of the material resistance passed. I had undergone a transformation facilitated by my experience. From frustration to willingness to try again.

The National Trust (2020) suggests that 'those who do nature-based activities are more likely to say they are happier than the rest of the population . . . [and] that everyone needs nature as a source of comfort in an uncertain world'. Robinson (2017) writes:

> When it comes to beefing up your happiness, it's hard to do better than engaged play. Not only does it align you with your deepest needs and deliver fun in the moment, but the social component of play is a huge predictor of increased daily well-being.

The National Trust proposes a number of ways we can engage playfully with nature, particularly in woodland spaces where all the senses can be refreshed and, in the next case-story, Patrick Boxall eloquently makes the connection between being 'at play' in nature and the nurture of creativity as an act of self-will.

Box 6.4 A second spring: growing creativity in the outdoors

Patrick Boxall

Lord Ancrum's Woods – roots that go back to the last ice age but gardened by the Lothian family, are now open as a place of quiet and discovery. Yew, giant sequoia, oak, birch, and Caledonian pine. Newbattle Abbey College, once for devotion and meditation, now for adult learning, creativity, and community. A Forest College. A place for living, where lives change.

Everyone comes to the woods. Seven ages in one place, time collapses into woodland time. The kindergarten, the schools, the students, the community, the volunteers. The remarkable thing is that they all want to do similar things – explore, climb, find, and always, always . . . make . . .

dens, fire, carvings, art, food, stories. There seems to be something fundamental about how folk play outdoors.

They tend to come into the woods in the spring, when the wild garlic is coming out, first fresh green, then that sharp smell underfoot, the flowers white by May. Tom is one of many, who come to claim something lost or, more often, something they knew was always there, but had forgotten how to find. 'Too old to climb trees', Tom is back at college after a winter that had left cracks and burns. Mistakes made, paths lost, heavy weather blowing through. A second spring, after many winters.

'Where is Tom?'
(In the cradle of a yew tree, 12 feet up, Tom is writing.)
'Come down, you're making me nervous!'
(He came down, smiling, to build a fire.)

Later, sitting, feeding and poking embers, talk moved around:

'I used to do this when I was wee . . . this was my childhood – making dens . . . I camped then . . . just in the woods . . . It was different then . . . Now I take my kids to the woods when they come to me for the weekends'.

Tom quietly showed me his poem. We make bread on the fire, with wild garlic, cooked on an old iron pan.

'I feel calm here'.

There is something about the woods that invites making. Being in the woods is to be creative: the blind office worker who led in making shelter; the department head who built a home for the wee folk; the man who wrote poems in the trees; the young man carving gifts for his gran; folk telling stories of creatures, trees, and streams. There are always stories – myths, imagined and remembered. Self-willed activity in self-willed land.

I talked to those who lead learning in the woods, about what it was like, what it meant, this creativity in the forest. Folk talked about people making and remaking, ideas of freedom, autonomy, play. Always relationships with place and person. Always voices making problems and possibilities. Always talking about some kind of justice for the people and the place, a justice for the human within the natural. Something about time and memory, connecting to who we were and what we could become.

A friend, a leader, hair as white as the garlic flowers, explained what it meant to her: 'Some people have an inner child, I have an outer child'.

The nuthatch is nesting in the hollow pine, the wood anemones are blooming, spring is here again; summer is coming. Late, but it is coming.

Finding a rhythm

Csikszentmihalyi (1999: 5) states that 'creativity presupposes a community of people who share ways of thinking and acting, who learn from each other and imitate each other's action' and that 'it is the community and not the individual who makes creativity manifest' (*ibid*.: 16). Play in nature offers both personal freedom and a sense of belonging – to the earth and to a community of others with whom we share our place on the earth. Ramblers (2020), a charity which aims to 'protect the ability of people to enjoy the sense of freedom and benefits that come from being outdoors on foot', promotes the social engagement and sense of comradery that comes from walking together in the natural environment – a rhythmic and synchronous activity with wide-ranging benefits for health and wellbeing (Hanson and Jones 2015). Zaraska (2020: 65) advocates the benefits of such synchronized activities, which can range from simple finger tapping in sync, to rowing as part of a crew, and singing in a choir – indeed any activity that involves simultaneous and coordinated movement, generating a 'complicated interplay . . . [which] results from a combination of neurohormonal, cognitive and perceptual factors'. Synchronous behaviors are also more likely to trigger endorphin systems, creating positive feedback loops that reinforce pleasure as well as relieving physical and mental pain (Zaraska 2020).

Another route to creativity is music-making. Paterson (2019) describes music as 'fundamental to being human' because it is 'emotionally satisfying like nothing else'. This sense of emotional satisfaction can be explained by the link between music and the release of the brain chemical dopamine (Levitin 2007), which is involved in the regulation of our moods and behavior, coupled with an increase in the pain-relieving effects of endorphins (Dunbar et al. 2012). This wellspring of neurochemicals explains why music makes us feel good and connected to other people. An investigation of the neural mechanisms underlying interpersonal synchrony (Kokal et al. 2011) supports the hypothesis that it is the rhythm in music which helps us to sync our brains and coordinate our body movements with others, increasing a sense of community and prosocial behavior. This tendency to synchronize seems to become even more important as we grow through the lifespan (Lang et al. 2015). A study by Nusbaum and Silvia (2010) found that people high in openness to experience are most likely to play a musical instrument, and Craft (2001) reported that graduates from music programs find that the creativity, teamwork, communication, and critical thinking developed in the course of their training are valuable and necessary life skills, regardless of their choice of occupation. Collective music-making seems to be both a natural resource for social cohesion and a fast-pass to creativity.

However, as in many other learning situations, the pressure to achieve – whether self-imposed or as a result of external demands and expectations – can interfere with the creative process when music-making becomes a source of frustration and anxiety rather than pleasure. The next case-story by Emilie Capulet describes a playful strategy for restoring the confidence of young musicians in a game of musical creativity.

Box 6.5 Watch for the laughs! The music of graphic scores

Emilie Capulet

The notation of music can be understood to be both the graphic and the symbolic representation of the sound of the music it represents. Amongst the different types of notation, two distinct approaches can be found: on the one hand, scores which include the traditional Western notational norms (staves, clefs, note values, rhythms, and associated musical symbols) as well as more unconventional graphic scores which strictly codify the composer's unique and personal take on music notation through specific instructions to performers as to how to read the score, and on the other hand, scores which feature uncodified visual analogues representing the music and giving the performers immense freedom and a more intuitive approach to an indeterminate and inherently ambiguous performance. The former can be quite prescriptive from an interpretative perspective, whilst the latter offers an open-ended multiplicity of interpretative outcomes. There are as many versions of a graphic score as there are performances of it.

A graphic score could be easily mistaken for a work of art, a sketch, a picture, a cartoon. One thinks here of the scores of Cathy Berberian, Tom Phillips, Györgi Ligeti, or Christian Wolff. In some cases, it resembles a technical diagram or a science project, such as Cornelius Cardew's *Treatise*, or the scores of Carl Bergstrøm-Nielsen and Martin Loyato, to name just a few, but all graphic scores reveal their musical essence in the way (musical) time coalesces with (graphic) space. Graphic scores are images which we apprehend in time, and that's what makes them inherently musical.

Musicians are usually well versed in reading traditionally notated scores, but when my university music students are confronted with a graphic score, their initial response is usually bewilderment and surprise leading to mirth and laughter as they try to make sense of the colors, the lines, and the patterns on the page.

Unlike traditionally notated scores, graphic scores do not have a long performance tradition. An uncodified graphic score puts the onus for the creation of the music entirely into your own hands. Anybody can play such a graphic score, in fact, even untrained musicians on unconventional instruments. What is important here is the personal approach and response to the image and the process of musical creation (see Figure 6.3 for an example of a graphic score by Emilie Capulet). My students, young adults at the threshold of their professional careers, were regularly suffering from intense anxiety in the pressure to perform set repertoire to what is considered to be the highest technical and musical standards of the competitions they were participating in. When given the task to play a graphic score, they started to forget their anxieties and channel their inner child in a game of musical creation, a game which they had long forgotten how to play as they progressed in their musical education and the stakes had got higher. To help these students approach all their music-making with the same positive and playful mindset, I then reversed the graphic score process as I asked them to draw the music they were going to be playing in their exams. They then each played each other's graphic scores to reveal the creative process going into each performance.

These playful musical and graphic activities led the students to gain confidence, musicality, and originality in their playing as they started to own their performances. One student felt that playing graphic scores was 'a freeing and relaxing experience' that had 'playfulness and freedom for sure. One which I think any musician could enjoy.' As Cornelius Cardew jotted down in his diary on 5 February 1965, with reference to his graphic score *Treatise*, 'watch for the laughs'!

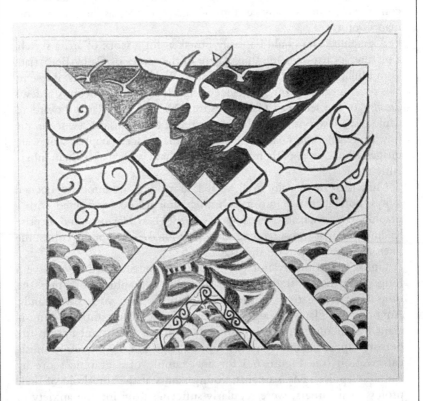

Figure 6.3 'Quartet', a graphic score by Emilie Capulet

Source: Photograph of an original drawing by Emilie Capulet.

This case-story highlights the importance of laughter as a natural mechanism for overcoming obstacles to creative practice. There is a growing body of literature linking the benefits of laughter and humor to improvement in various aspects of our personal and professional development. Humor as a character strength facilitates many positive outcomes, such as positive emotions and positive relationships (Ruch et al. 2019). Gonot-Schoupinsky et al. (2020) examine the link between laughter and health, including its positive impact on sleep, anxiety, and depression and the role of humor and laughter in self-care and integrative medicine. Berk (cited in Gonot-Schoupinsky et al. 2020) discusses how humor, when it induces laughter, produces biochemical changes and analgesic qualities which can relieve stress, tension, and fear providing an antidote for the complexity of modern life which increases during early adulthood as work and family commitments take center stage. As we have seen, humans, unlike most other species, continue to play into adulthood and have done so throughout history and across cultures (Neale 2020). The presence of play in adulthood reflects our innate capacity to learn, to adapt, and to thrive throughout the lifespan, as we evolve culturally as well as biologically (*ibid.*).

Playing for love: dancing to a new tune

The song and dance of attachment and separation which begins at the start of life, and then assumes a new guise in adolescence, is transformed once again with the move to adulthood. When a young person leaves home – to study, work, or travel – both they and their parents undergo 'a massive plastic change, as they alter old emotional habits, routines, and self-images' (Doidge 2007: 117). As the emergent adult enters this new developmental stage, their play also assumes a new shape and meaning as the drive to form new intimate attachments takes priority. Freeman (1999) has argued that forming a romantic attachment in early adulthood demands a process of neuronal reorganization during which oxytocin – the trust hormone – serves to liberate the young adult from earlier attachments, leaving them free to learn new patterns of connection. Panksepp (1998) offers the complementary view that it is oxytocin's role in reducing separation-distress which frees the young adult to form new bonds while reconfiguring existing relationships.

It has long been established that a playful disposition is related to many positive outcomes – such as lower stress (e.g., Barnett 2011); more positive interactions with other people (Proyer 2014); creativity (e.g., Glynn and Webster 1992); physical fitness (Proyer et al. 2018); and overall wellbeing (Proyer 2013). It is now also becoming clear that play also has a positive role in our most intimate adult relationships (Proyer and Brauer 2019).

At the start of a romantic relationship, play and playfulness again become crucial mediators of attachment. Traces of childhood play reemerge in the lovers' use of baby talk, gentle teasing, and delight in 'naughty' behavior between the bedsheets (Doidge 2007). Ablon (2001) identifies three points of commonality between adult play and that of children – exploration, imagination, and amusement – stating that 'the play of adults serves to promote development, awareness, organization, and mastery of affect' (*ibid.*: 346) in a continuation of the process of personal growth and adaptation.

One of the first definitions of the intimate play that takes place between romantic partners was provided by Betcher (1977: iv), who described it as 'private language, sexual foreplay, wrestling and tickling, and various forms of joking and teasing'. Klein (1980: 75) subsequently added to this definition, summing up adult playfulness as 'a joyous expression of a state of well-being'. As at the start of life, intimate playfulness fulfills the human attachment needs for safety, comfort, and connection and represents that 'safe place' where the individual can reveal their authentic selves (*ibid.*).

Proyer et al. (Proyer and Brauer 2019) conducted a study to examine the link between playfulness and positive emotion, communication, relationship satisfaction, and happiness in couple relationships. They differentiated between four types of playfulness (other-directed, lighthearted, intellectual, and whimsical) and found that the couples in their study tended to share a similar play style. Couples sharing an 'other-directed' play style (such as jocular teasing or playful interaction) and those with an 'intellectual' play style (such as problem-solving and playing with ideas) each reported greater relationship satisfaction, an optimistic outlook, and more sexual satisfaction. Proyer et al. (*ibid.*) concluded that 'playfulness is important in romantic life', perhaps because it 'may facilitate positive experiences in relationships and help couples embrace the lighter side of life' (*ibid.*).

Our understanding of the positive impact of playfulness on relationship quality rests on the observation that being playful 'allows people to frame or reframe everyday situations in a way such that they experience them as entertaining, and/or intellectually stimulating, and/or personally interesting' (Proyer 2017). Playfulness stimulates positive emotions (e.g., joy, interest, connection, and love) which in turn have a wide-ranging influence on personal wellbeing (Fredrickson 2001). Positive emotions not only build future resilience but also increase the likelihood that an individual will experience more positive emotions in the future – what Fredrickson calls a 'positive upward spiral'. This may account, at least in part, for the correlation which has been identified between playfulness, physical activity, and health-motivated behaviors (Proyer et al. 2018).

Playfulness is also associated with flexible thinking, which is a fundamental aspect of psychological health and may also contribute to physical wellbeing and an active lifestyle (Kashdan and Rottenberg 2010). It may be that the association between a playful disposition and the flexibility to adapt to change is a key indicator of desirability in romantic attachments. De Koven (2015) references the theory 'that play and the personal characteristic of playfulness, among adult humans, send signals, or messages, to the opposite sex of important information regarding the signaler's suitability as a long-term mate' (Chick et al. 2012) suggesting that adult play may actually be a 'survival skill', because it nurtures the flexibility of thought and behavior that helps us to respond and adapt to change.

From lover to parent

Bandura's (1986) theory of reciprocal determinism has helped psychologists to understand that who we become and the choices we make in life result from the symbiotic relationship between our personal characteristics and the environment in which we grow. In the long-running debate about the balance of influence between our biological inheritance (nature) and our social experiences (nurture), James (2017) argues that human relationships are primarily determined by parenting rather than genetics. This is a perspective which has been widely criticized (e.g., Plomin 2019), but there is a general acceptance that the developmental process both influences and is influenced by our environment from conception onwards. It follows that our play history from the start of life will play a part of deciding how we adapt to the role of parent.

The transition from being part of a couple to becoming parents involves one of the most profound reorganizations of the lifespan, with changes in the brains, endocrine systems, behaviors, identities, and relationships of everyone involved (Divecha 2015). It is a transition which requires a shift in the attachment relationship away from the satisfaction of personal needs to providing protection, comfort, and care for a child. A wealth of research has shown that our own experience of parental attachment impacts on the ways we think, feel, and behave in the context of romantic relationships (Mikulincer and Goodman 2006). John Bowlby (1988), the father of attachment theory, predicted that a parent's own attachment experiences and representations would subsequently influence their attitudes and behavior when they became parents themselves. Studies have shown that adults who are identified as having a secure attachment to their own parents tend to be more sensitive and responsive parents themselves and to have a positive (secure) attachment relationship with their own children (van Ijzendoorn 1995). In a recent review of the literature, Jones et al. (2015) found compelling evidence for an association between parents' self-reported attachment styles and many aspects of parenting, including parents' thoughts, feelings, and behavior in relation to their parenting role.

The transition to parenthood is often associated with a dip in relationship satisfaction (Rauch-Anderegg et al. 2019). There may be a decline in the quality and quantity of communication, and the reality of family life rarely matches the expectations fostered by the glossy images of family life portrayed in the media (Cowan and Cowan 1988). Sleepless nights, practical demands, and financial pressures can make it hard for new parents to relax enough to enjoy each other's company, be flirtatious, humorous, and playful. Yet, a playful disposition can facilitate communication and problem-solving, serves as a pressure release valve, and boosts morale (Csikszentmihalyi 1992). If we accept the premise that play is about growth and adaptation to change in one's social and emotional environment (Sutton-Smith 1997), the rediscovery of play in early adulthood can ease the transition from romantic coupling to parenthood and family responsibilities.

The past decade has been characterized by advances in the application of digital technology, including the rapid expansion of the video gaming industry which is now accessed by an estimated third of the world population (Neale 2020). Young adults have now overtaken children and adolescents as the primary consumers of video game content (Patterson and Barratt 2019), and interactive gaming is an increasingly popular adult playground. For young parents who experience an abrupt curtailing of their social life with the arrival of children, playing video games online with adult peers can restore a feeling of social belonging. Barlett et al. (2008) have suggested that game-playing in adulthood may represent an escape from problems, rather than being a cause of them and, when not used to excess, video games can have positive effects on wellbeing (Neale 2020). In the final case-story of this chapter, Carla Roberts describes how becoming part of an online gaming community has addressed the social isolation so often experienced by young parents, increasing her sense of trust and confidence, and enabling her to develop interpersonal skills which can be applied to other areas of her life.

Box 6.6 And mummy plays too: finding friendship in the world of online gaming

Carla Roberts

I have enjoyed playing video games from an early age, and this didn't change with the transition from child to adulthood. I dabbled in a few online games, but it was only when a friend invited me to join him in playing *Final Fantasy XIV* that I began to delve deeper into the world of MMOs (*Massively Multiplayer Online games*). I found it intimidating at first, knowing that millions of other players could see my virtual character and interact with me; however, playing alongside a friend I had known for more than ten years, I quickly gained in confidence. We joined a 'Free Company' together (a group of people in-game who interact socially and help each other progress through the game) and this opened the door to 'voice chat'.

Talking directly with other players over various platforms, it soon became clear that the relationships formed in-game could extend into real life. Within a matter of weeks, I was part of a group of people who I would speak to on a daily basis. Knowing that these were people with the same interests as me, removed the limitations you might find when meeting new friends in real life. There was no need to create a false façade or to pretend to want to see people when I just wanted to sit at home in front of the TV. If I wanted to speak to people, I could log in, and when I wanted to stop, I would log out.

Having a young child to raise by myself, this social interaction proved invaluable to me: it was on my own terms, and I could fit it around my son when it suited him – and all from the comfort of my own home. There was no need for a military operation to arrange a babysitter with a time limit on how long I could stay out. I could sit at home in my pyjamas with a cup of tea, having an actual social life, while my son slept soundly in the next room. These online friendships soon spilled over into real life and I no longer needed to be logged into the game to engage with them. We connected over various social media sites, exchanged phone numbers, and over time got to know everything about each other – probably more than with a lot of the friends I had in real life.

After nearly three years of speaking to each other every day, we all decided to meet up for real and, when we got together, it was just like getting together with old friends. I came to see these people as real friends, not just a group of strangers who happen to play the same video game. We had arguments, we made up, we shared secrets, photos, and special moments in our lives and when two of the group got married, we all met up for a second time. It is now nearly five years since we had that first awkward conversation over voice chat, and I can safely say these 'play-mates' are a huge part of my life for good.

Conclusion

Early adulthood is an important life stage because it is the last opportunity to acquire the mental capital and build the cognitive reserves which will be drawn upon in later life. With maturation of the brain complete, relative neural stability allows for the emergence of a period of creativity and innovation in both the personal and professional domains. Play is one way in which we explore and experiment, create and innovate, to 'transform the familiar into something new and exciting' (Neale 2020: 31). This readiness to adapt and change is crucial to the formation of close relationships and family life as we learn to care for others as well as ourselves. Adulthood is described as 'a golden age' for play because of the human capacity to learn and adapt across the lifespan, and because 'when we play, we thrive too' continuing the process of biological and cultural evolution (*ibid.*).

References

Ablon, S. L. (2001) Continuities of tongues: A developmental perspective on the role of play in child and adult psychoanalytic process. *Journal of Clinical Psychoanalysis*, 10: 354–365.

All Party Parliamentary Group on Arts Health and Wellbeing (2017) *Creative Health: The Arts for Health and Wellbeing: The Short Report*. London: All Party Parliamentary Group on Arts Health and Wellbeing.

Bandura, A. (1986) *Social Foundations of Thought and Action: A Social Cognitive Theory*. New Jersey: Prentice-Hall.

Barlett, C. P., Anderson, C. A. and Swing, E. L. (2008) Video game effects: Confirmed, suspected, and speculative: A review of the evidence. *Simulation & Gaming*, 40 (3): 377–403.

Barnett, L. A. (2011) How do playful people play? Gendered and racial leisure perspectives, motives, and preferences of college students. *Leisure Sciences*, 33: 382–401.

Betcher, R.W. (1977). *Intimate play and marital adaptation: Regression in the presence of another* (Doctoral dissertation, Boston University). Dissertation Abstracts International, 38, 1871.

Bowlby, J. (1988) *A Secure Base: Parent-Child Attachment and Healthy Human Development.* London: Routledge.

Brown, S. (2008a) *Why Play Is More Than Just Fun.* Online. HTTP: <www.ted.com/talks/ stuart_brown_play_is_more_than_just_fun#t-464084> (accessed 19 March 2020).

Brown, T. (2008b) *Tales of Creativity and Play.* Online. HTTP: <www.ted.com/talks/tim_ brown_tales_of_creativity_and_play/transcript?language=e> (accessed 19 March 2020).

Center on the Developing Child (2020) *Brain Architecture.* Online. HTTP: <https:// developingchild.harvard.edu/science/key-concepts/brain-architecture/> (accessed 26 September 2020).

Chick, G., Yarnal, C. and Purrington, A. (2012) Play and mate preference testing the signal theory of adult playfulness. *American Journal of Play*, 4 (4): 407–440.

Christensen, T. (2014) *Why Play Is Essential for Creativity.* Online. HTTP: <https:// creativesomething.net/post/84134598535/why-play-is-essential-for-creativity> (accessed 19 March 2020).

Coast (2016) *What Happens to Your Brain after 25?* Online. HTTP: <www.thecoast.net.nz/ shows/days-with-lorna-subritzky/what-happens-to-your-brainafter25/#:~:text= Your%20brain%20is%20now%20also,believe%20is%20a%20genuine%20phenomenon> (accessed 26 September 2020).

Cowan, C. P. and Cowan, P. A. (1988) Who does what when partners become parents. *Marriage and Family Review*, 12 (3–4): 105–131.

Craft, A. (2001) *An Analysis of Research and Literature on Creativity in Education.* Online. HTTP: <www.creativetallis.com/uploads/2/2/8/7/2287089/creativity_in_education_report. pdf> (accessed 28 September 2020).

Csikszentmihalyi, M. (1992) *Flow: The Psychology of Happiness.* London: Random House.

Csikszentmihalyi, M. (1999) *A Systems Perspective on Creativity.* Online. HTTP: <www. sagepub.com/sites/default/files/upm-binaries/11443_01_Henry_Ch01.pdf> (accessed 24 March 2020).

Csikszentmihalyi, M. (2013) *Creativity: The Psychology of Discovery and Invention.* New York: Harper Perennial.

Cummins, E. (2017) *3 Life-Changing Things That Happen to the Human Brain at 25.* Online. HTTP: <www.inverse.com/article/33753-brain-changes-health-25-quarter-life-crisis-neurology> (accessed 26 September 2020).

Deary, I., Corley, J., Gow, A., Harris, S., Houlihan, L., Marioni, R., Penke, L., Rafnsson, S. and Starr, J. (2009) Age-associated cognitive decline. *British Medical Bulletin*, 92 (1): 135–152. https://doi.org/10.1093/bmb/ldp033.

De Koven, B. (2014) *A Playful Path.* Online. HTTP: <Lulu.com>.

De Koven, B. (2015) Playfulness is a survival skill. Online. HTTP: <www.aplayfulpath. com/playfulness-is-survival-skill/> (accessed 10 March 2020).

Dinishak, J. (2016) The deficit view and its critics. *Disability Studies Quarterly*, 36 (4). Online. HTTP: <https://dsq-sds.org/article/view/5236/4475> (accessed 26 September 2020).

Divecha, D. (2015) *The Transition to Parenthood: What Happened to Me?* Online. HTTP: <www.developmentalscience.com/blog/2015/11/30/the-transition-to-parenthood-what-happened-to-me> (accessed 29 September 2020).

Doidge, N. (2007) *The Brain That Changes Itself*. New York: Penguin.

Dunbar, R. I., Kaskatis, K., MacDonald, I. and Barra, V. (2012) Performance of music elevates pain threshold and positive affect: Implications for the evolutionary function of music. *Evolutionary Psychology*, 10 (4): 688–702.

Elkind, D. (2007) *The Power of Play*. Cambridge, MA: Da Capo Press.

Foresight Mental Capital and Wellbeing Project (2008) *Systems Maps*. London: The Government Office for Science.

Fredrickson, B. L. (2001) The role of positive emotions in positive psychology: The broaden-and-build theory of positive emotions. *American Psychologist*, 56: 218–226.

Freeman, W. J. (1999) *How Brains Make Up Their Minds*. London: Weidenfeld and Nicolson.

Glynn, M. A. and Webster, J. (1992) The adult playfulness scale: An initial assessment. *Psychological Reports*, 71: 83–103.

Gonot-Schoupinsky, F., Garip, G. and Sheffiled, D. (2020) Laughter and humour for personal development: A systematic scoping review of the evidence. *European Journal of Integrative Medicine*, 37, August. doi.org/10.1016/j.eujim.2020.101144.

Hannah, M. (2014) *Humanising Healthcare: Patterns of Hope for a System under Strain*. Dorset: Triarchy Press Ltd.

Hanson, S. and Jones, A. (2015) Is there evidence that walking groups have health benefits? A systematic review and meta-analysis. *British Journal of Sports Medicine*, 49: 710–715.

Huizinga, J. (1955) *Homo Ludens: A Study of the Play Element in Culture*. Boston, MA: Beacon Press.

Inspiring Scotland (2016) *Loose Parts Play*. Online. HTTP: <www.inspiringscotland.org.uk/wp-content/uploads/2017/03/Loose-Parts-Play-web.pdf> (accessed 19 March 2020).

James, O. (2017) *Not in Your Genes: The Real Reasons Children Are Like Their Parents*. London: Vermilion.

Jones, J. D., Cassidy, J. and Shaver, P. R. (2015) Parents' self-reported attachment styles: A review of links with parenting behaviors, emotions, and cognitions. *Personality and Social Psychology Review*, 19 (1): 44–76.

Kashdan, T. B. and Rottenberg, J. (2010) Psychological flexibility as a fundamental aspect of health. *Clinical Psychology Review*, 30: 865–878.

Klein, D. B. (1980) Playfulness in marriage: A psychoanalytic perspective. *Dissertation Abstracts International*, 41: 693.

Kokal, I., Engel, A., Kirschner, S. and Keysers, C. (2011) Synchronized drumming enhances activity in the caudate and facilitates prosocial commitment – if the rhythm comes easily. *PLoS ONE*, 6 (11): e27272.

Korn, P. (2013) *Why We Make Things and Why It Matters*. London: Vintage.

Lang, M., Shaw, D. J., Reddish, P., Wallot, S., Mitkidis, P. and Xygalatas, D. (2015) Lost in the rhythm: Effects of rhythm on subsequent interpersonal coordination. *Cognitive Science*, 40 (7): 1797–1815.

Lawton, G. (2009) *The Five Ages of the Brain: Adulthood*. Online. HTTP: <www.newscientist.com/article/mg20227023-000-the-five-ages-of-the-brain-adulthood/> (accessed 26 September 2020).

Levitin, D. J. (2007) *This Is Your Brain on Music: The Science of a Human Obsession*. New York: Penguin.

Mikulincer, M. and Goodman, G. S. (Eds.) (2006) *Dynamics of Romantic Love: Attachment, Caregiving, and Sex*. New York: Guilford Press.

National Trust (2020) *Everyone Needs Nature*. Online. HTTP: <www.nationaltrust.org.uk/features/everyone-needs-nature> (accessed 27 September 2020).

Neale, D. (2020) A golden age of play for adults. *The Psychologist*: 28–31.

Nusbaum, E. C. and Silvia, P. J. (2010) Shivers and timbres: Personality and the experience of chills from music. *Social Psychological and Personality Science*, 2 (2): 199–204.

Panksepp, J. (1998) *Affective Neuroscience: The Foundations of Human and Animal Emotions*. New York: Oxford University Press.

Paterson, L. (2019) *Never Mind the Maths, Music Needs to Blow Its Own Trumpet*. London: The Sunday Times.

Patterson, T. and Barratt, S. (2019) *Playing for the Planet: How Video Games Can Deliver for People and the Environment*. Arendal, Norway: UN Environment/GRID-Arendal.

Perry, G. (2014) *Playing to the Gallery*. London: Penguin.

Pink, D. H. (2007) *A Whole New Mind: Why Right-Brainers Will Rule the Future*. New York: Riverhead Books.

Plomin, R. (2019) *Blueprint: How DNA Makes Us Who We Are*. London: Penguin.

Proyer, R. T. (2013) The well-being of playful adults: Adult playfulness, subjective well-being, physical well-being, and the pursuit of enjoyable activities. *European Journal of Humour Research*, 1: 84–98.

Proyer, R. T. (2014) Playfulness over the lifespan and its relation to happiness: Results from an online survey. *Zeitschrift für Gerontologie + Geriatrie (Z Gerontol Geriatr)*, 47 (6): 508–512.

Proyer, R. T. (2017) A new structural model for the study of adult playfulness: Assessment and exploration of an understudied individual differences variable. *Personality and Individual Differences*, 108: 113–122.

Proyer, R. T. and Brauer, K. (2019) *Playfulness in Romantic Relationships: Is Love Really Such an Easy Game to Play?* Online. HTTP: <www.spsp.org/news-center/blog/proyer-brauer-playfulness> (accessed 9 March 2020).

Proyer, R. T., Gander, F., Bertenshaw, E. J. and Brauer, K. (2018) The positive relationships of playfulness with indicators of health, activity, and physical fitness. *Frontiers in Psychology*, 9: 1440.

Ramblers (2020) *Our Mission*. Online. HTTP: <www.ramblers.org.uk/about-us/what-we-do/our-mission.aspx> (accessed 27 September 2020).

Rauch-Anderegg, V., Kuhn, R., Milek, A., Halford, W. and Bodenmann, G. (2019) Relationship behaviors across the transition to parenthood. *Journal of Family Issues*, 41 (4): 483–506.

Richards, M. C. (1989) *Centering in Pottery, Poetry, and the Person*. Middletown, CT: Wesleyan University Press.

Robinson, J. (2017) *The Key to Happiness: A Taboo for Adults?* Online. HTTP: <www.huffingtonpost.com/joe-robinson/why-is-the-key-source-of-_b_809719.html> (accessed 28 September 2020).

Ruch, W., Platt, T., Proyer, R. T. and Chen, H.-C. (2019) *Humor and Laughter, Playfulness and Cheerfulness: Upsides and Downsides to a Life of Lightness*. Lausanne: Frontiers Media SA.

Russ, S. W. and Kaugars, A. S. (2010) Emotion in children's play and creative problem solving. *Creativity Research Journal*, 13 (2): 211–219.

Sass, L. A. (2001) Schizophrenia, modernism, and the 'creative imagination': On creativity and psychopathology. *Creativity Research Journal*, 13 (1): 55–74.

Saunders, R. (2020) *Finding a Slice of Creativity during a Global Pandemic*. Online. HTTP: <www.japantimes.co.jp/life/2020/05/31/lifestyle/zen-bread-coronavirus/> (accessed 26 September 2020).

Simonton, D. (2001) *The Psychology of Creativity: A Historical Perspective*. Online. HTTP: <https://simonton.faculty.ucdavis.edu/wpcontent/uploads/sites/243/2015/08/HistoryCreativity.pdf> (accessed 19 March 2020).

Stiegler, B. (2010) *Taking Care of Youth and the Generations* (S. Barker, Trans.). Stanford: Stanford University Press.

Sutton-Smith, B. (1997) *The Ambiguity of Play*. Cambridge, MA: Harvard University Press.

van Ijzendoorn, M. H. (1995) Adult attachment representations, parental responsiveness, and infant attachment: A meta-analysis on the predictive validity of the adult attachment interview. *Psychology Bulletin*, 117 (3): 387–403.

Warner, S. A. and Myers, K. L. (2009) The creative classroom: The role of space and place toward facilitating creativity. *Technology Teacher*, 69: 28–34.

Weinberg, B. A. and Galenson, D. W. (2019) Creative careers: The life cycles of Nobel laureates in economics. *De Economist*, 167: 221–239.

Wilson, J. (2017) *Creativity in Times of Constraint: A Practitioner's Companion in Mental Health and Social Care*. Oxon: Routledge.

World Health Organization (2020) *Constitution*. Online. HTTP: <www.who.int/about/who-we-are/constitution> (accessed 26 September 2020).

Zaraska, M. (2020) All together now. *Scientific American*, 323 (4): 64–69.

7 The middle years

According to the Cambridge Dictionary (2020), middle age is 'the period of life, usually considered to be from 45–60 years of age when you are no longer young but are not yet old'. Carl Jung (2001: 140) called the middle years 'the afternoon of life' and it is often thought of as a lull between the dynamism of adolescence and early adulthood and the slow amble into old age. However, Lachman et al. (2015) construe this period as a pivotal point, 'linking childhood experiences with midlife health and lifestyle in midlife with health in old age' (Lachman 2015: 6). At an interpersonal level, adults in their middle years influence the wellbeing of younger generations through their roles as parents, caregivers, and mentors, while their own wellbeing is similarly influenced by the circumstances of those around them (*ibid.*). As such 'the midlife falls at the crossroads of gains and losses for many aging-related processes and life domains' (*ibid.*: 6).

By the age of 45, the physical maturation process is complete, and the changes associated with aging become increasingly apparent. Physical health and functioning have passed optimal levels; there are the first signs of a decline in sensory sharpness and the onset of chronic health conditions (Liberty University n.d.). Although there is some commonality between the sexes, in relation to decreases in physical strength and functioning, there are also gender-specific changes (*ibid.*), many of which are linked to hormonal influences, which trigger specific changes in the brain (Brizendine 2007, 2011).

However, the reality for many people is that the middle years are a positive time of life with many advantages: a heightened sense of freedom and control; peace of mind; self-awareness; and self-acceptance (Dolberg and Ayalon 2017). While it is commonly believed that brain activity slows down with age, recent studies have overturned this assumption, suggesting that the middle-aged brain not only preserves many of the capacities of youth, but it also acquires new potential (e.g., Reuter-Lorenz and Park 2010). Four or five decades of experiential enrichment are reflected in 'an enduring potential for plasticity, reorganization and preservation of capacities' (Reuter-Lorenz cited in Phillips 2011). Perhaps, the most striking feature of the middle years is the wide variation in physical, mental, and social health at this time of life.

There is a dearth of research into middle age (Lachman 2015) but increasing acknowledgment of the importance of the middle years for health in later life, particularly in relation to the maintenance of cognitive reserve (Age UK 2020) and the prevention of ill-health and disability. Steel et al. (2018) advocate the prioritization of effective primary prevention strategies, since lifestyle choices taken by the age of 45 will influence our chances of living longer, happier lives at both an individual and societal level (Cabinet Office and Department of Health and Social Care 2019). Reuter-Lorenz (cited in Phillips 2011) advises that, 'middle age should be thought of as a time for a new form of self-investment' because it 'brings so many new opportunities to invest in your own cognitive and physical resources, so you can buffer against the effects of older age'. This is where play, with its emphasis on creativity, innovation, and enjoyment, coupled with its restorative and self-reinforcing benefits, can make a real difference.

A time for work, rest, and play

'Play matters, no matter how old you are' (Hirsh-Pasek, cited in Keller 2017), but as we become established in our adult lives – as partners, parents, and workers – play can take a back seat. There has been a growing awareness in recent years of the value of adult 'play-time' for physical and mental wellbeing (Tonkin and Whitaker 2016), as well as for work performance and productivity (Petelczyc et al. 2018), but making time for play amidst the hustle and bustle of daily life presents some obvious challenges. As far back as 1970, Linder identified that 'the desire and ability to consume [leisure] would increase more rapidly than the time available to do so', creating 'the now widespread feeling that life has become more pressured, and [explaining] why people feel busier than ever before' (Haworth and Roberts 2008: 4).

Work–life balance is the term used to describe the state of equilibrium in which equal attention is devoted to one's work life, family life, and personal life – including time for rest and play. In the UK, workers fare badly on international comparisons of work–life balance, ranking 24 out of 25 comparable economies (Chartered Institute of Personnel and Development 2019). Three out of five UK employees report working longer hours than they would like to, a condition exacerbated by home working which can blur the boundaries between work and everything else (*ibid.*). While UK workers tend to perceive work as having a positive impact on their physical and mental health, it is also cited as a source of physical and mental stress for a significant proportion of the workforce. Two in five UK workers report having experienced a work-related health condition in the previous 12 months – typically musculoskeletal, anxiety, and sleep problems (*ibid.*) – with significant consequences for personal and public health (Public Health England 2019).

Research by the Office for National Statistics [ONS] (2013) indicates that how people view their health is one of the most important factors contributing to overall personal wellbeing. In the last decade, there has been a decrease in self-reported health in the UK, suggesting that more people believe themselves to be in worse health, despite World Health Organization (2020) estimates that, on average, we are living longer, healthier lives over this period (ONS

2019). A survey by the Health and Safety Executive [HSE] (2019) found that over 600,000 workers suffered from work-related stress, depression, or anxiety in 2018–2019, resulting in almost 13 million working days lost due to ill-health. The HSE reports that 44 per cent of all cases of work-related ill-health is due to mental health problems, which account for 54 per cent of all working days lost due to ill-health. It is perhaps unsurprising that those working in public service industries (such as health, education, and social care) report the highest levels of stress (*ibid.*).

Wilson (2017: 37) acknowledges that 'when we are caught up in repetitive and unproductive processes in our work, it is easy to see how we become disillusioned and resigned to follow the increasing demands on our energy and willingness to continue to do a good job' with negative consequences for both job satisfaction, worker morale, and collective wellbeing. Play promotes novelty and behavioral flexibility in both animals and humans (Bateson and Martin 2013), and as a source of behavioral variety it stimulates divergent thinking, legitimizing the search for new ways of working which better support health and wellbeing in the workplace. A survey by the Chartered Institute of Personnel and Development (2020) found that 89 per cent of organizations which had introduced activities to improve the health and wellbeing of the workforce reported positive outcomes, in terms of morale, engagement, and a more inclusive culture.

The following two case-stories describe the benefits to health and wellbeing when play and playfulness find their way onto the 'shop floor'. They illustrate the positive impact of social contagion when play is encouraged and celebrated through the co-creation of play-space in the course of the working day. In the words of Daniel Pink (2008: 188), 'play is emerging from the shadows of frivolousness and assuming a place in the spotlight'.

Box 7.1 Satsuma Fridays and mindful play: caring for carers using mindfulness techniques

Gavin Cullen

Friday and the atmosphere in the nurses' duty room was tense. Kate, Mary, and John, experienced Child and Adolescent Mental Health Service nurses, looked exhausted. They were silent, disconnected from each other, focusing on computer screens. That week, Kate had been involved in supporting a young person with suicidal intentions, while Mary and John had been called to help someone who had barricaded themselves into their bedroom during a family row. About half the client group had experienced a crisis of one sort or another. As team leader, I felt that we needed a lift and to reconnect. Kate had recently disclosed a talent for juggling, so I asked the team to stop working and invited Kate to teach us – using the only obvious thing to hand . . . satsumas.

Following initial grumbling reluctance, the group began to focus on this new, perhaps strange and, for me, challenging task. Mindfulness involves being aware of present moment experience with curiosity and kindness, as opposed to shutting down some experiences, because they feel unpleasant for example, or berating ourselves for the way we do things (Choden and Regan-Addis 2018). Satsuma juggling definitely qualifies as a technique for practicing those qualities, as I learned when I misjudged a juggle, and a satsuma burst open on my forehead. The group energy had already begun to change, the juggling allowing space to open up between us and our worried, tired thoughts and feelings. But in this moment, we also just had a good laugh.

Now, nursing is a serious business, as are all forms of caring, and rightly so. Nursing involves engaging with, and trying to alleviate, human suffering and its causes. Enemies to that purpose, at least in mental health practice, include mindless caring routines and tasks; being overly certain or fixed in our thinking; and taking the burden of suffering onto our own shoulders. Hawkins and Shohet (2007) remind us that our job as carers is to create the space within which change is possible, rather than take full, personal responsibility for change. Mindfulness not only helps create space, but it can also freshen our perspectives and re-energize us. We cannot pour from empty cups.

Mindfulness too can be a bit serious. And I don't just mean the images of young, slim, attractive people sitting in annoyingly perfect postures we see everywhere on social media. Meditation practice of any kind can be hard graft (Kaiser Greenland 2016). We need to play in and with mindfulness practice too. As a mindfulness teacher, one game I recommend for use in mindfulness training is: *first letter, last letter* (Miller et al. 2017). It's simple: I say a word, and then the next person says a word that begins with the last letter of my word, and so on. Easy, right? In my experience, for round one only. Go slightly quicker for round two, and a playful chaos commences. Mistakes are made and the natural comedy of being human in groups emerges.

Go on, try it! We all need a Satsuma Friday from time to time.

Box 7.2 Work at play: yoga with healthcare workers

Lorraine Close

It goes without saying that the wellbeing of healthcare professionals is of paramount importance in healthcare. Yet doctors and nurses have higher rates of burnout, stress, and depression than the general population (Dyrbye et al. 2017). This is a global trend that literature has shown impacts on job satisfaction, patient safety, and empathy (*ibid.*).

The issues that impact on the mental wellbeing of health professionals are complex, often at a political or organizational level, related to staffing or resources. There is increasing pushback against a discourse that promotes 'responsibilization' or individual responsibility for improving wellbeing and denies organizational or political responsibility (Traynor 2018). This can mean that activities that promote self-care and wellbeing can feel tokenistic or patronizing to healthcare workers when offered as a means of encouraging relaxation or wellbeing. This is something which must be acknowledged when developing staff wellbeing programs.

In NHS Lothian, Edinburgh Community Yoga has been working on staff wellbeing programs since 2014, offering yoga-based programs as a means to explore self-care, and how self-care can help to contribute to 'micro cultures' or organizations that promote and support wellbeing. These initiatives started as 30-minute psychoeducation programs and now run as eight-week wellbeing programs incorporating yoga, mindfulness, psychoeducation, reflective practice, and crucially, fostering a sense of a community or group that promotes and supports wellbeing. We bring people together to make small and appropriate changes in their own behavior and to begin to foster a workplace that values, supports, and creates wellbeing. Practicing yoga brings us to the present moment. It helps us to develop a sense of self-compassion, stillness, and an acceptance of that which we cannot control. We learn to breathe and remember what relaxation feels like. Creating this space allows people to notice how they are feeling and to consider how things could be different.

> '*I feel calmer and more rested by the end of the week even although the workload hasn't changed. I generally feel I have more energy and have used the breathing techniques to calm myself during times of pressure. It also made me more aware of triggers for others in my team, which helped me offer support and take action, ultimately getting the best from them*'.

Yoga doesn't have to look the way it does on social media. When we practice yoga with healthcare staff it looks like tired doctors and nurses just sitting in a chair breathing for ten minutes. It looks like overworked medics contemplating when was the last time they made time for themselves to do something they enjoy and then writing down how they might make time for the one thing that brings them joy, charges their batteries, and reminds them who they are outside of their jobs.

> '*This workshop has made me realise I haven't done anything for years. How can I support my junior doctors to be well when I don't even know how to be well myself?*'

We are all somebody, and we are all more than one thing. Remembering this in a society that favors success and specialty over balance and happiness can be challenging. Our NHS staff wellbeing workshops give people the opportunity to literally stop and notice, to move and to breathe, and to reconnect with what they love; to remember that looking after yourself is not self-indulgent but in fact necessary to remain effective care-givers and compassionate healthcare professionals and, importantly, individuals who have meaning in life outside of work.

Ways to wellbeing

Wellbeing is a multidimensional concept which is about more than just the absence of health problems and involves a balance between physical, psychological, social, and economic variables. The ancient Greek principle of *eudaimonia*, which describes a state of health, happiness, and prosperity, is encapsulated in the World Health Organization's definition of wellbeing as 'an ability to realize personal potential, cope with daily stresses, and contribute productively to society' (Corkhill et al. 2014: 34).

Modern life involves a complex tapestry of roles and responsibilities, and the associated maelstrom of external pressures can be overwhelming. Sjöberg and Porko-Hudd (2019: 49) describe a 'life entangled and entwined due to expectations and demands from work, family and friends as well as from social media'. Evidence suggests that playful participation in creative arts and crafts can act as a counterbalance to the busyness of day-to-day life, helping 'to untangle [the] demanding situations' (*ibid.*) which can precipitate mental or physical health problems.

The New Economics Foundation (2011) produced a set of evidence-based public mental health messages known as the *Five Ways to Wellbeing*: Connect, Be Active, Take Notice, Keep Learning, Give. These messages reflect behaviors that can be adopted by anyone, to improve or maintain their wellbeing and mental health, and they link with play in various and often surprising ways. The following case-story by Kathrine Jebsen-Moore, for example, illustrates how these 'Five Ways' find expression in the simple art of knitting.

Box 7.3 Knitting: playing with colors, textures, and shapes to create something useful

Kathrine Jebsen-Moore

I was not a natural-born knitter. When I learned to knit at school, I was among the slowest and most uneven knitters in my class. I still have one of the first things I knitted: a crooked teddy-bear made with coarse, pink wool. It was not until I was expecting my first child that I became seriously interested in the craft; I managed to knit a blanket and a hat for him, while outsourcing the more complicated garments to my mother. But I gradually became more engrossed in the craft: I bought my first pattern book, which has been almost used up by now and is falling apart at the seams and started to plan what I wanted to make. Thinking of color combinations and choosing the patterns became an important part of my new hobby.

'Really, all you need to become a good knitter are wool, needles, hands, and slightly below-average intelligence. Of course, superior intelligence, such as yours and mine, is an advantage', says legendary knitter Elizabeth Zimmermann (1971), the woman behind the iconic 'baby surprise jacket'. I agree with Zimmermann's sentiment: in generations past, almost everyone could knit. Even my grandfather, as a little boy in Norway, taught himself to knit a pair of mittens one winter when his mother was too busy. Knitting only requires one to learn a few basic stitches, and once you know how, all you need is patience and practice. When I meet someone who admires my handiwork, they often say, 'I wish I could do that!', and I tell them that, if I can, anyone can.

Knitting is not just a pleasurable pastime with which to fill your time, whether you are traveling, listening to the radio, or watching children in the playground – although it is a very satisfactory way of doing so as, by the end, you can easily see your progress. It's also a sensory experience, as you move from the original idea – perhaps browsing the countless patterns now available online, or designing your own project on paper – to deciding on your yarn – wool, alpaca perhaps, or cotton with linen for a summer garment? – to casting on. As you knit, you might stop to feel and look at the fabric as it flows from your needles, albeit slowly, and you picture the finished product in your mind. Once it's done, there is excitement in trying it on – whether it's for yourself or perhaps a child – and hopefully pleasure as you see that it fits well. And to dress yourself or your child, or maybe a good friend, in something you've made from a long piece of string, gives you confidence and pride.

Knitting is no longer something we do because we have to, as it's often cheaper, and of course easier and much quicker, to buy readymade garments. But for me, knitting time is play time, while still being a sensible, productive activity which leaves you feeling that not only have you enjoyed yourself, but you have made use of otherwise 'dead' time. It can be a welcome distraction when you're feeling stressed, and an outlet of nervous energy that otherwise would go to waste. To quote Elizabeth Zimmermann again (and I recommend her if you really want to explore the art of knitting): 'Properly practiced, knitting soothes the troubled spirit, and it doesn't hurt the untroubled spirit either'.

The Greek meaning of the word *rhythm* is to flow (Project Resiliency 2020), and the therapeutic rhythm of knitting is just one example of how a creative activity can nurture a state of 'being well' (Corkhill 2014). Another example of rhythmic play is drumming, which offers a whole brain workout and can 'induce deep relaxation, lower blood pressure, produce feelings of wellbeing [and] release emotional trauma and reduce stress' providing 'support [for] individuals, families and communities in times of joy, sadness and change' (Project Resiliency 2020). Drumming has been a part of human culture since ancient times, as a form of communication and ritual celebration. Playing with others as part of a 'Drum Circle' nurtures social connectedness by alleviating unhealthy preoccupation with the self and reducing feelings of social isolation and alienation (*ibid.*).

Playing together: physical activity and social connection

In Ancient Greece, play and physical exercise were inseparable (Andreu–Cabrera et al. 2010), and observations of the play of young children throughout history reveal that it is typically a lively, active process (Whitaker 2019). Play and physical activity share a symbiotic relationship: we are more inclined to play when we are feeling well; and play nurtures a sense of wellbeing which induces us to engage in health-giving behaviors (Proyer 2013). It is well established that the physical aspects of play have a positive impact on mental health by reducing anxiety, depression, and negative mood and by improving self-esteem and cognitive function (Sharma et al. 2006). In their book *Spark!* Ratey and Hagerman (2010: 245) make the case that physical activity 'has a profound impact on cognitive abilities and mental health. It is simply one of the best treatments we have for most psychiatric problems'.

Numerous studies have shown that children engage in active, physical play when they perceive it to be enjoyable (e.g., Brockman et al. 2011). However, adults seem to lose their sense of joyful, physically active play and, in adulthood, physical activity tends to assume primarily functional purposes. Thiel et al. (2016: 14) make the point that 'for adults fun and wellbeing appear to be not an essential part of their physical activity' and suggest that reframing physical activity in the context of play and 'fun' may be a way to engage individuals in physical activity with all the associated benefits for holistic health, as shown in Figure 7.1. Corkhill (2014: loc 189) proposes that 'people need to want to be active before you can succeed in getting them active mentally and physically, so a preliminary stage which stimulates interest, desire and motivation is crucial for successful involvement in managing health and wellbeing'.

De Koven (2014) speaks of 'reclaiming' our health through play, an idea inherent in the following case-stories which illustrate how physical activity which is embedded in a social network is one of the most beneficial health pursuits (Smith and Christakis 2008).

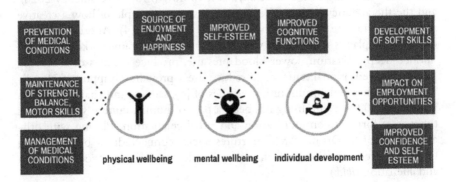

Figure 7.1 Wider role and benefits of physical activity

Source: (Public Health England 2020) reproduced under Commons Creative Licence 3.0.

Box 7.4 Wheelchair basketball: finding the fun in physical exercise

Claire Weldon

We all know that physical exercise is good for us, but it can often feel like hard work, something to tick off the list before getting on with the things we want to do. The NHS recommends that adults engage in some type of physical activity every day, and at least 150 minutes of moderate-intensity activity each week (NHS 2019). I have a physical disability which makes this hard to achieve. I understand the health benefits of exercise so make myself do it but, at times, I find my trips to the gym dull and monotonous.

One morning, as I walked reluctantly through the sports hall at the leisure center, on my way to the gym, I noticed two women around my own age taking part in a wheelchair basketball coaching session. I stopped to watch, and it looked fun so I asked if I could join them – and from that moment I was hooked.

I am now part of a small group of people who attend wheelchair basketball training sessions twice a week: on a Tuesday evening after work and before work on a Thursday. We are of various ages, sizes, and shapes, and some of us have disabilities or medical conditions. However, once we are in a wheelchair, our differences are irrelevant. Wheelchair basketball is the first sport I have tried, in which I can participate on equal terms as everyone else.

Aspire Leisure Centre, where the coaching takes place, is the 'first leisure centre in Europe for disabled and non-disabled people' (Aspire 2020). Because of the nature of the center, a wide variety of people attend, including children, adults, and older people. Some have disabilities or health conditions, but many do not. The leisure center is in the grounds of a hospital, so it is not unusual to see all sorts of people there: no one 'bats an eyelid' about how someone walks or talks or what they wear.

Our wheelchair basketball sessions incorporate a wide range of activities, including wheelchair skills and circuit training as well as basketball. I have experienced huge benefits from attending the sessions. I have developed core strength, wheelchair skills, and basketball skills, such as hand–eye coordination and been able to participate in cardiovascular exercise. While none of us are likely to turn professional, we are improving our basketball skills as well as our strength and stamina. We do not play in a league and certainly do not take ourselves seriously, but one thing is for sure – we do have a lot of fun!

Taking part in the wheelchair basketball training is also good for my mental health: I look forward to attending the coaching sessions, which have become an important part of my week. Friendships and support networks have developed alongside the physical benefits: we support each other when one of us has had a difficult hospital appointment or is feeling unwell and meet regularly for a drink and a chat to catch up on each other's news. We have an active WhatsApp group, which we use to arrange coaching sessions and also to share news and jokes.

For the first time in my life, I have found that it is possible to enjoy physical exercise, despite having a disability and being over the age of 40. Taking part in wheelchair basketball has allowed me to find the fun in exercise, while benefiting my physical, mental, social, and emotional health. It is something that I hope to continue with for as long as possible.

Box 7.5 Playful engagement through social media: #NHS1000miles and Parkrun

Kath Evans

From my experience, social media can embrace a playful approach to human connection and engagement with others . . . let me share my story.

It was a Sunday afternoon, the sun was streaming through the patio doors as my friendly neighbor Anna took me under her wing and introduced me to the Twitter-sphere, just one of a range of digital engagement tools. She was an expert teacher and skillfully helped me to navigate the process of creating a profile and a personal biography, educated me on the use of images, and encouraged the creation of lists of influencers, whilst offering hints and tips on building a network and advice on maturing connections. That sunny afternoon represented the start of many happy, inspiring, and playful years of social connection in a digital landscape. As the years have passed, through playful trial and error, I have gained confidence and maturity in navigating this virtual world.

Social media has also had an impact on my wellbeing and engagement with physical playfulness. In the autumn of 2017, I was seeking inspiration to celebrate and amplify the seventieth birthday of the NHS. Using Twitter, a few of us explored whether it would be possible to enhance our physical health by covering 1000 miles during the course of a year, and in doing so to give the NHS a birthday gift of us not needing to use it – as far as possible! It became clear that the evolving community wanted the challenge to be an inclusive one so, however they were achieved (swimming, walking, running, cycling) they would all count toward the 1000 miles annual target.

In 2018 the community of #NHS1000miles was born, with a blog using a simple word press tool offering supportive guidance. The Sunday evening 7.30 p.m. 'tweet meet' provided a weekly check in, an opportunity to share pictures of activities and mileage totals, using the hashtag #NHS1000miles to collate the tweets. The buzz of Twitter activity continues years after the original challenge was completed, offering inspiration and encouragement to continue playful physical activity, and at the end of each year the mileage clock is reset.

Lisa, an NHS Leader, has reflected on the loss of a dear friend during the first year of #NHS1000miles: the challenge encouraged her to get out into nature each week to build up her miles, creating time and space to remember a wonderful friend as she tromped the fields in the knowledge that she could check in with the Twitter community on Sunday evening. This playful, supportive #NHS1000miles community has encouraged people to take a daily walk, even try out their local ParkRun, an initiative started by Paul Sinton-Hewitt in 2004 to encourage people to complete 5K on a Saturday morning. As a result of this Twitter support, I have become an ultra-runner (an ultra-run is any distance beyond that of a marathon, 26.2 miles). It's been quite a journey!

I have found that social media can embrace a playful approach which is also purposeful, nurturing an inclusive culture through community engagement. The currency of social media is engagement. Our behaviors drive impact, digital listening, content creation, compilation, and summarizing of activities and can lead to enhanced physical and emotional wellbeing in what is an ever-expanding digital world.

Creative approaches to mental health

The most widely quoted research suggests that one in four people in the UK experiences a mental health problem during the course of a year, with one in six experiencing mental distress in any given week (McManus et al. 2016). The incidence of poor mental health is highest within the working-age population and affects women more than men (Cabinet Office and Department of Health and Social Care 2019). However, these statistics need to be treated with caution (Mind 2020), and myths of a global mental health epidemic have been refuted: 'All the modeling we've done in high-income countries where there is survey data which has tracked over time shows that the prevalence hasn't changed – it's flatlined' (Whiteford cited in Rice-Oxley 2019).

What has changed in relation to mental health in recent years is an increased recognition of the functional impact of mental health problems and of the range of effective treatment options. While antipsychotic medication remains the first line of treatment worldwide, feeding a global market worth an estimated 80 billion dollars per annum (BCC Research 2014), there is a growing body of research indicating natural, low-cost, low-impact alternatives to drug treatment. Clinical evidence for the effectiveness of non-pharmacological interventions for a wide range of health problems has spurred the drive for *social prescribing*, or community referral, which is reflected in an ambition to make 'play on prescription' available to one million people in England by 2023–2024 (Cabinet Office and Department of Health and Social Care 2019). The National Academy for Social Prescribing (2020a: 3) describes social prescribing as 'discovering or rediscovering the joy in life, trying something new, or building on a hidden or long forgotten talent' to enable people to 'live the best life they can'. Marie Ann Essam (cited at National Academy for Social Prescribing 2020b) is quoted as saying, 'Social prescribing represents the most effective, wide reaching and life changing of all initiatives in my 30 years as a GP'.

The effectiveness of creative and playful approaches to preventing and treating mental distress is supported by the evidence that therapeutic activities which are experienced as enjoyable are the most effective (e.g., Pizarro 2004). A report by the All-Party Parliamentary Group [APPG] on Arts Health and Wellbeing (2017) found that self-motivated participation in creative activities can promote, preserve, and restore mental health, supporting 'longer lives, better lived' (Slawson 2017). A systematic review of art therapies supports this observation, concluding that 'art therapy appears to have statistically positive effects compared with controls in a number of studies in patients with different clinical profiles' (Uttley et al. 2015). In the words of artist, Grayson Perry: 'a world without art is an inhuman world. Making and consuming art lifts our spirits and keeps us sane' (cited in APPG 2017).

The following case-stories describe two different approaches to 'lifting the spirits' through creative endeavors.

Box 7.6 Art, identity, and the return to wellness

Nisi Conyngham

Make-up has been used by humans throughout our history for effect in beauty, rituals, theatre, film, fashion, and sub-cultures. Children paint their faces as they experiment with different personas and their associated emotions. Make-up is a human art form that has been influenced by culture, as well as by society and politics, a personal flow of creative expression which gives rise to a sense of self and form to cultural identity.

Over a quarter of a century ago, I embarked on a career in make-up artistry, initially working freelance on weddings and editorial shoots and, in time, teaching other people skills in this art form. Through my work I began to witness the positive effects make-up had on an individual's confidence as well as on a group's collective ability to develop their sense of creative self-expression.

As I grappled with chronic severe depression and anxiety, I subconsciously drew on my creative practice in make-up artistry to look inwards. It was during this time that I truly came to understand the capacity held by make-up as a healing art. I began to tread new territory, with a fresh creative direction, as I progressed from working solely on the face, to painting the body. Demanding concentrated focus, it is mentally and physically exhausting but, in the flow of the moment, also deeply rewarding. Through body art, I tentatively, slowly, discovered a safe way to communicate and process my thoughts, emotions, and beliefs.

As my mental health declined, and as I tried to overcome the insurmountable loss of self-identity, disconnection, and dissociation from internal and external worlds which followed a suicide attempt, I took the concept of working with the body to another level. Working with my own body, I chose to communicate my self-concept in a triptych which represents my soul, body, and mind and my disconnection from each. With assistance, I painted different colors onto my body, each brush stroke primal, textured in its application, symbolizing the different emotions and spiritual meanings related to each aspect of the soul, body, and mind. The depth and texture were enhanced through post-editing. At times, the creative process was emotionally fraught, filled with doubts and insecurities. However, I was also able to explore and actualize the true intentions behind this artwork; to give each thought, emotion, and experience an identity of their own; a voice of their own; and a home of their own in order to live outside of me. Trapped as they are within the confinements of a photographic image (Figure 7.2), I am now able to see my past experiences separate from who I am. They have shaped me but do not define me. The ritualized painting of my face and body reunited my connection to this life, to my body, to my mind, and to my soul, giving rise to a restored sense of self. This is the healing power of make-up as art.

I do not underestimate the importance of 'Timeless Time' and how creating it provided closure to a dark chapter in my life, but it also acted as a catalyst for change, enabling me to look outwards; connecting me to the wonders of the natural world through the creative practices of photography and botanical art.

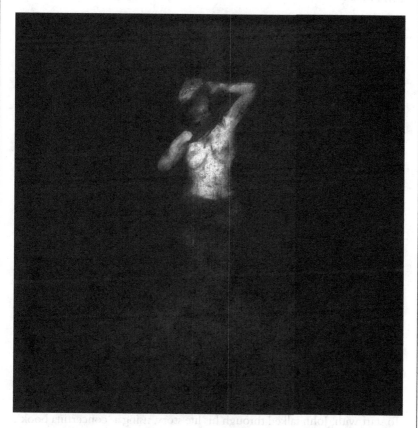

Figure 7.2 The Body, 'as it dissolves into the shadows, so does my connection to it'

Source: Photograph by Leigh Bishop Photography.

Since its inception in 1969, Garvald Edinburgh, has been creating 'community through creativity' by helping people with learning disabilities 'to express their creativity, to find meaning in work, and to feel part of a community'. It is an approach which recognizes 'the uniqueness of each person and their hopes, aspirations and contributions . . . supporting them to feel valued, make friends and learn new skills' (Garvald Edinburgh 2020). In the next case-story, Eric Fleming describes a co-working relationship which reflects these principles.

Box 7.7 Creating a social play space: making room for meaningful biographies

Eric Fleming

From the early 1990s I worked in various roles at Garvald Edinburgh, an organization inspired by the ideas of Rudolf Steiner and the principles of Social Therapy (Garvald Edinburgh 2018), and, until recently, I worked for 20 years as group leader in the Glass Studio.

In 2018, I was invited to deliver a working group on the theme of *'Social Play Space: Making Room for Meaningful Biographies'* at the Goetheanum International Conference (Fleming 2018). I submitted a proposal to co-run this working group with John, a member of the Glass Studio who has learning disabilities. The intention was for workshop participants to explore their life stories and to express these visually in the form of a three-dimensional artistic book. Steiner describes seven-year phases which punctuate our lives; understanding how these unfold in our own life stories enables us to also understand the life stories of others, thus building bridges between people (Burkhard 2002).

Before inviting John to co-lead this workshop, I had to consider what he might gain from the experience. It felt important to engage him in all stages of the planning process; deciding how we would structure the workshop and what our different roles would be. We both needed to feel confident that John would be able to share his personal history and his artistic abilities without becoming overwhelmed. John is naturally drawn toward creative activities with others, he is a talented maker, and he loves to learn about other people; a workshop on the themes of play and biography presented an ideal opportunity for him to build confidence through a meaningful focus in guiding and supporting others.

The working group included 18 participants from around the world. To start with, John talked through his life story, using a 'concertina book'. This is a freestanding book in three-dimensional form and is often created with an emphasis on textures and images (Figure 7.3). Using the example of John's own book, along with other similar samples, we invited participants to think about how they might create their own 'life story book'.

We then led the group in an artistic game which involved smaller groups of 3–4 people being given a box of miniature objects (including people, animals, insects, shells, feathers, hearts, gemstones), which they selected one by one and used to build a group narrative to later share with the whole group. This game was a 'building process', designed to encourage participants to flex their ability to recall their own narrative over time and to find a way to relate this in a meaningful way. Symbolism can be a 'safe' way to express difficult themes or experiences, spelling them out in a personal or visceral way. Storytelling is an imaginative and playful way to convey meaning and may allow for deeper insight into how critical moments in life have been negotiated or been consequential (Kearney 1997).

After this game, John and I demonstrated the different ways in which art and craft materials could be used by the participants to make a concertina book of their own life stories. John demonstrated various printing techniques and we jointly supported people as they started work on their own projects. John has a disarming smile, infectious giggle, and a playful nature which he expresses in humorous banter and gentle teasing. His relaxed and easy manner put participants at ease, enabling them to engage confidently with the various aspects of the workshop in a spirit of social playfulness.

To close the workshop, John led another exercise in which participants were asked to draw themselves as a young plant. They were invited to add to each other's drawings with the image of something (such as rain or sunshine) that would be nurturing to the new growth.

When designing activities for people with learning disabilities, play and playfulness are often used to enliven interest and involvement. I witnessed John thrive and shine in his role as workshop leader; he was happy, relaxed, and buoyant throughout the whole experience. Play has a role in many therapeutic and educational endeavors because of its potential for overcoming barriers to meaningful engagement, such as communication challenges, lack of motivation, low self-esteem, or lack of confidence. These are barriers which any of us might come up against in life, and play can be the key that opens the door to autonomy and choice, which are the bedrocks of a healthy life (Fleming and Whitaker 2019).

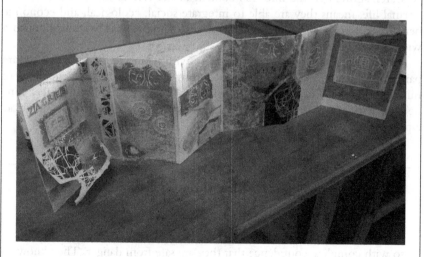

Figure 7.3 A concertina life story book

Source: Photograph by Eric Fleming.

The case-stories discussed here demonstrate the importance, for both personal and public health, of *mental health literacy*, '[whereby] everyone has the skills, knowledge and confidence to improve their mental health and wellbeing throughout life' (Cabinet Office and Department of Health and Social Care 2019: 40). The human mind has the remarkable ability to positively reframe difficult experiences, something Grayson Perry (2014: 108) describes as an 'amazing survival mechanism [which] can often translate the most harrowing brutalities into masterpieces that speak to us all'.

Natural healing

Since ancient times, healers have advocated the importance of nature for health. The concept of 'ecotherapy' has evolved from this tradition, which frames human health and wellbeing in the context of the health of the earth and its natural ecosystem (Summers and Vivian 2018). Exercise in nature (e.g., Gladwell et al. 2013); horticultural therapy (e.g., Cameron 2020); forest-bathing (Ling 2018); animal-assisted therapy (Fine 2019); and even views of the natural environment (e.g., Raanaas et al. 2011) have been cited as having a positive impact on both physical and mental wellbeing.

Care farms, such as Pathways in Suffolk in the UK, which engage vulnerable people in farming or horticulture activities as a form of therapy have been shown to enhance wellbeing and self-esteem and provide a sense of community (Pathways Care Farm 2020) through a combination of social interaction, physical activity, and connection with nature. In the Netherlands, which has four times as many care farms as the UK, they are regarded as healthcare institutions. Research shows that the informal context of the care farm, which is close to normal life, means they are able to integrate social, ecological, and economic benefits and go beyond meeting the needs of individuals to contribute to a wider health culture (Hassink et al. 2020).

Finding a connection, or reconnection, with nature reminds us that we are part of the planet, rather than separate from it and incorporates elements of mindfulness and of deep play. A readiness to embrace the playful fosters connection with place, with others, and with 'the creative, social, and political' aspects of the self (Warburton 2017).

Box 7.8 Safe to play. Healing through horticulture

Jan Cameron

When I watch my four-year-old twin granddaughters playing, they do so with complete confidence that they are safe from danger. They know the rules and that their safety and behavior is monitored by their mother in whom they have complete trust. They do not check for any oncoming threat and they are completely free to get absorbed in what they are doing. They do not think about what they look like and have no notion at all of being judged. So deep is their absorption in their play they will not hear me calling them.

How can we recreate these conditions for adults with a history of trauma? Is our ability to play and enjoy humor a measure of how safe and comfortable we feel?

In the garden –

George always appeared anxious, head bowed low, and became paralyzed when asked to make the simplest decision – "Would you like tea or coffee?" "Would you like to take a book home?"

I watched him one day as he was looking on at the others who were involved in a game of "hedge surfing", where they took turns to hurl themselves at a leylandii hedge that was due to come out. He was a picture of misery and longing. I asked him if he would like to join in and he said no, but that it looked fun. I sat with him a while and he haltingly explained that he was frightened that if people saw him 'having fun' and 'playing' they would stop believing how bad he felt and would think he had been exaggerating and consequently drop his support.

Growing up, he had spent many years being judged and told he had no reason to be unhappy when he felt truly miserable, and he did not trust his own feelings. He did eventually join in the fun, but not that day. He gradually came to see, through watching others playing, that there was a place for play, even when people were deeply anxious or depressed. It was ok to look as if you were enjoying yourself, not worry about what other people might think, and just be silly for a little while. Once people start having fun, recovery is a real possibility.

I never understood why people always seemed to want to do the jobs I thought were awful – like dragging boulders out of the river and pulling them up the hill into the garden to make a rockery? I would ask for volunteers, not feeling hopeful, and six hands would shoot up. Then, when you came to watch them doing it, it was all about play! They loved it – splashing in the water, soaking each other, dropping the stone halfway up the hill and watching it roll back down, laughing and starting again; making friends, forgetting all their troubles, and for a few minutes becoming completely absorbed in the task. Working together they got to know each other. Reliving it all and talking about it afterwards over tea. People who normally really struggled to talk to anybody.

It takes real courage to play when you live your life in fear, but it opens a window just for a few minutes onto what it might feel like to be well.

The family that plays together . . .

The Modern Families Index 2019 (Working Families 2019), which examines the relationship between work and family life, found that only a quarter of those surveyed thought they had achieved the right balance for family wellbeing. Almost 50 per cent of parents felt that work had impacted negatively on the time they spent with their partners and/or children. They reported that work impinged on their ability to exercise (47 per cent), to eat healthily (43 per cent), and on their sleep pattern (47 per cent).

The power of play is trans-generational, and it has been shown that families who play together enjoy a happier and healthier lived experience of 'family', regardless of socio-economic circumstance or individual characteristics (Cohen 2008). A UK study (Hill 2010) reported that 20 per cent of parents say they have forgotten how to play with their children, while 55 per cent of children want more play time with their parents and grandparents. Multigenerational play offers psychological and health benefits for parents and offspring alike, including reduced stress, improved mood, superior cognitive skills, and enhanced relationships (Fromberg and Bergen 2006), as illustrated by our next two case-stories.

Box 7.9 Taking to the hills: rediscovering joy in the outdoors

Julia Findon

My first hill walks were with my parents at the age of 11. I accepted that this was just what we did on holiday and have no memory of either enjoying or hating it – but I did love the scenery and had a fascination for lakes and mountains.

After achieving my Duke of Edinburgh Gold award (DofE 2020) at the age of 20, hiking was replaced with studies, career, marriage, and children, and – even though I maintained an interest in the outdoors through my involvement with the Scout Association (Scouts 2020) – I didn't take to the hills again until I was 46. By then, our family had acquired a dog and I had started taking him on longer walks close to home, reviving memories of childhood trips to the Lake District. I wondered if a return visit would live up to my treasured memories and decided to ask one of my sons (then 16 years old) if he would like to go to the Lakes with me. Fortunately, he agreed and we both loved it, although we never imagined where that exercise in mother–son bonding would lead.

The two of us, plus the dog, started going to either Snowdonia or the Lakes at least once a year and, while I was happy to plod up and down a mountain, Rob's teenage ambitions took off and soon he was rock-climbing and seeking out new challenges. In 2010, he persuaded me to undertake the National Three Peaks Challenge (2020), climbing the three highest peaks in the UK within 24 hours. This was followed a year later by a trip to Africa to climb Mounts Kenya and Kilimanjaro and, two years after that, we conquered Mont Blanc followed by a winter climbing course in Scotland.

Rob pushed me into each new challenge, and I am so glad he did as I never imagined I could meet any of them. Rob is now a qualified Mountain Leader and, in his role as a teacher, he runs numerous outdoor trips for his students.

I now spend most of my holidays in the Lake District: hillwalking, scrambling and, if Rob can join me, we go climbing together. Mostly, the dog and I walk on our own and I am quite happy up in the hills with just my own company. There is always something new to discover and the hillwalking fraternity are a diverse and friendly crowd. But I love it best of all when one – or better still both – of my sons want to walk with me, allowing for some real quality time.

Recently, my eldest grandson has started joining us on our expeditions – three generations taking to the hills together. The mountains are our family playground, providing calm, beauty, solitude, and togetherness – and, when least expected, the thrill of an adrenaline rush.

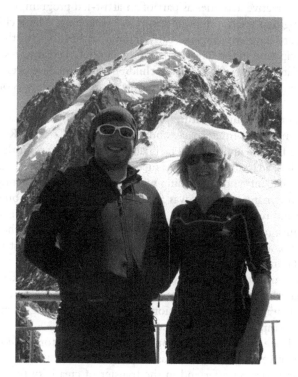

Figure 7.4 Julia and Rob at Petite Aiguille Verte

Source: Photograph by Julia Findon.

Box 7.10 Creative Kin: a collaborative play-based approach to support for kinship carers

Starcatchers

When a child cannot be looked after by their own parents, they are most likely to go to live with a family member or adult friend who knows them well. This arrangement, whether formal or informal, is known as Kinship Care and it is estimated that between 11,000 and 16,000 children in the UK are looked after in this way (Kidner 2016). Providing kinship care is an act of generosity, but it presents significant practical, social, and emotional challenges for everyone involved. In the words of De Koven (2015) 'It's not such an easy thing to do, remembering to have fun' – especially when life is hard'.

Creative Kin was a two-year pilot project delivered to kinship care families in partnership between *Children 1st*, Scotland's national children's charity, and Scotland's national arts and early years organization, *Starcatchers*, between 2017 and 2019. Kinship care families in two areas of Scotland were given the opportunity to explore music, visual art, drama, and other creative activities as part of an artist-led program, designed to help strengthen relationships and improve wellbeing. Many children in kinship care have experienced early trauma within their birth families, and participation in the Creative Kin project offered creative respite from the associated stresses, both for the children and for their carers, with the space to enjoy quality time together away from the challenges of day-to-day life.

One of the defining features of play is that it is a fluid state, varying in form across time, space, and context. The Creative Kin project adopted a flexible approach to facilitating creative play with the kinship care families, adapting themes and media to reflect the interests and needs of the participants and responding with sensitivity to a constantly changing group dynamic. 'There was focused, energetic facilitation – always listening and reacting, with the aim of keeping attention, satisfying creative whims, responding to creative wishes, going with what the children brought up, and adding new ideas in a persuasive way' (artist reflection cited in Grant and Morton 2019: 11).

Evaluation of the Creative Kin project highlighted three key benefits emerging from this approach. First, it provides kinship families with both the opportunity and the permission to simply have *fun* together, separate from the complications and difficulties of daily life.

Second, the creative play sessions inspired participator *confidence* in the use of creative media, which was reflected in a commitment to shaping the activities on offer and in the transfer of creativity to other areas of their lives. This corroborates De Koven's (2014: 150) assertion that 'playing seems to nurture the development of a whole vocabulary of skills and arts and social forms'.

Third, participation in the project strengthened *relationships* between the children and their kin, while also providing a platform for carers to share their own experiences with peers, and to be supported by the reassurance that they are not alone.

These three themes are identifiable in the example of a kinship carer who attended Creative Kin with her own two children and her child in kinship. High levels of stress within the home had created tensions between family members which could escalate to distressing levels, threatening the stability of the arrangement. Participation in the project offered opportunities for the children to play, share, and laugh together, as well as reducing the isolation of the carer through social contact with a peer group. Being part of Creative Kin showed the family that they could spend time together without getting into conflict and inspired the carer to use creative activities at home to continue to strengthen relationships. All family members demonstrated improvements in the self-regulation and self-compassion which are critical for building personal resilience.

The shared experience of play and laughter is known to trigger the release of the trust hormone oxytocin which acts as a 'social glue', promoting empathy and the sense of wellbeing that derives from being part of a positive interaction (Zak 2011). Creative Kin demonstrates how playful engagement in creative activities can bind families together and act as a stabilizer in uncertain times.

Conclusion

Play in adulthood may not always appear 'playful', but it merits the appellation because it incorporates all the defining features of play. First, play must be freely chosen and self-directed; motivated intrinsically rather than for external reward. Like the play of children, adult play requires imagination to set it apart from the reality of day-to-day life. It may be guided by mental rules, but flexibly so, and demands an alert and active state of mind, free from stress and open to possibility (Gray 2013: 274). Play ceases to be playful if the player participates under instruction to do so, but adults often need affirmation that their natural drive toward playfulness is not only permitted but encouraged, indeed celebrated. Play theorist and practitioner, Bernie DeKoven, states that

> the important thing for adults is to allow themselves to be playful. Because playfulness, like humor, is a survival skill. It helps us adapt to change, to engage each other, to create community. Playfulness is flexibility, responsiveness, openness, sensitivity, awareness. It connects us to life.
>
> (De Koven 2015: 145)

References

Age UK (2020) *Cognitive Reserve*. Online. HTTP: <www.ageuk.org.uk/information-advice/health-wellbeing/mind-body/staying-sharp/thinking-skills-change-with-age/cognitive-reserve/> (accessed 30 May 2020).

All-Party Parliamentary Group on Arts, Health and Wellbeing (2017) Online. HTTP: <www.culturehealthandwellbeing.org.uk/appg-inquiry/> (accessed 14 April 2020).

Andreu-Cabrera, E., Cepero, M., Rojas, F. J. and Chinchilla-Mira, J. J. (2010) Play and childhood in ancient Greece. *Journal of Human Sport and Exercise*, 5 (3): 339–347.

Aspire (2020) *Home*. Online. HTTP: <www.aspire.org.uk/> (accessed 21 April 2020).

Bateson, P. and Martin, P. (2013) *Play, Playfulness, Creativity and Innovation*. Cambridge: Cambridge University Press.

BCC Research (2014) *Drugs for Treating Mental Disorders: Technologies and Global Markets*. Online. HTTP: <www.bccresearch.com/market-research/pharmaceuticals/mental-disorder-drugs.html> (accessed 14 April 2020).

Brizendine, L. (2007) *The Female Brain*. New York: Bantam Books.

Brizendine, L. (2011) *The Male Brain: An Essential Owner's Manual for Every Man, and a Cheat Sheet for Every Woman*. New York: Bantam Books.

Brockman, R., Jago, R. and Fox, K. R. (2011) Children's active play: Self-reported motivators, barriers and facilitators. *BMC Public Health*, 11: 461. doi.org/10.1186/1471-2458-11-461.

Burkhard, G. (2002) *Taking Charge Your Life Patterns and Their Meaning*. Edinburgh: Floris Books.

Cabinet Office and Department of Health and Social Care (2019) *Advancing Our Health: Prevention in the 2020s: Consultation Document*. Online. HTTP: <www.gov.uk/government/consultations/advancing-our-health-prevention-in-the-2020s/advancing-our-health-prevention-in-the-2020s-consultation-document> (accessed 11 September 2020).

Cambridge Dictionary (2020) *Middle Age*. Online. HTTP: <https://dictionary.cambridge.org/dictionary/english/middle-age> (accessed 30 May 2020).

Cameron, J. (2020) *The Garden Cure*. London: Saraband.

Chartered Institute of Personnel and Development (2019) *UK Working Lives: The CIPD Job Quality Index*. Online. HTTP: <www.cipd.co.uk/Images/uk-working-lives-summary-2019-v1_tcm18-58584.pdf> (accessed 9 April 2020).

Chartered Institute of Personnel and Development (2020) *Health and Wellbeing at Work*. Online. HTTP: <www.cipd.co.uk/Images/health-and-well-being-2020-report_tcm18-73967.pdf> (accessed 8 May 2020).

Choden and Regan-Addis, H. (2018) *Mindfulness-Based Living Course*. Alresford, Hampshire: O-Books.

Cohen, L. J. (2008) *Playful Parenting: An Exciting New Approach to Raising Children That Will Help You Nurture Close Connections, Solve Behavior Problems, and Encourage Confidence*. New York: Random House.

Corkhill, B. (2014) *Knit for Health and Wellbeing: How to Knit a Flexible Mind and More . . .* [Kindle]. Bath: Flatbear Publishing.

Corkhill, B., Hemmings, J., Maddock, A. and Riley, J. (2014) Knitting and well-being. *TEXTILE*, 12 (1): 34–57.

De Koven, B. (2014) *A Playful Path*. Pittsburgh, PA: ETC Press.

De Koven, B. (2015) Deep fun and the theater of games: An interview with Bernie De Koven. *American Journal of Play*, 7 (2): 137–154.

DofE (2020) *Home*. Online. HTTP: <www.dofe.org/> (accessed 22 April 2020).

Dolberg, P. and Ayalon, L. (2017) Subjective meanings and identification with Middle Age. *The International Journal of Aging and Human Development*, 87 (1): 52–76.

Dyrbye, L. N., Shanafelt, T. D., Sinsky, C. A., Cipriano, P. F., Bhatt, J., Ommaya, A., West, C. P. and Meyers, D. (2017) *Burnout among Health Care Professionals: A Call to Explore and Address This Underrecognized Threat to Safe, High-Quality are.* NAM Perspectives. Discussion Paper. Washington: National Academy of Medicine.

Fine, A. H. (2019) *Handbook of Animal Assisted Therapy.* Amsterdam: Elsevier.

Fleming, E. (2018) *Social Play Space: Making Room for Meaningful Biographies.* Goetheanum International Conference, Dornach.

Fleming, E. and Whitaker, J. (2019) The art of public health and the wisdom of play: Participation in the creative arts as a route to health and wellbeing. In: Tonkin, A. and Whitaker, J. (Eds.), *Play and Playfulness for Public Health and Wellbeing.* Oxon: Routledge.

Fromberg, D. P. and Bergen, D. (2006) *Play from Birth to Twelve: Contexts, Perspectives and Meanings.* Abingdon: Taylor and Francis.

Garvald Edinburgh (2018) *Social Therapy Charter.* Online. HTTP: <www.garvaldedinburgh.org.uk/social-therapy-charter-16/> (accessed 21 November 2020).

Gladwell, V. F., Brown, D. K., Wood, C., Sandercock, G. R. and Barton, J. L. (2013) The great outdoors: How a green exercise environment can benefit all. *Extreme Physiology and Medicine,* 2: 3. doi.org/10.1186/2046-7648-2-3.

Grant, A. and Morton, S. (2019) *Starcatchers: Creative Kin Evaluation Report: Matter of Focus.* Online. HTTP: <www.starcatchers.org.uk/wp-content/uploads/2019/05/Matter-Of-Focus-Report-FINAL.pdf> (accessed 2 March 2020).

Gray, P. (2013) Play as preparation for learning and life. An interview with Peter Gray. *American Journal of Play,* 5 (3): 271–292.

Hassink, J., Agricola, H., Veen, E. J., Pijpker, R., de Bruin, S. R., van der Meulen, H. A. B. and Plug, L. B. (2020) The care farming sector in the Netherlands: A reflection on its developments and promising innovations. *Sustainability 2020,* 12: 3811. doi:10.3390/su12093811.

Hawkins, P. and Shohet, R. (2007) *Supervision in the Helping Professions.* Maidenhead, Berkshire: Oxford University Press.

Haworth, J. and Roberts, K. (2008) *State-of-Science Review: SR-C8 Leisure: The Next 25 Years.* London: The Government Office for Science.

Health and Safety Executive (2019) *Work-Related Stress, Anxiety or Depression Statistics in Great Britain, 2019.* Online. HTTP: <www.hse.gov.uk/statistics/causdis/stress.pdf> (accessed 16 April 2020).

Hill, A. (2010) *Parents Are Forgetting How to Play with Their Children, Study Shows.* Online. HTTP: <www.theguardian.com/lifeandstyle/2010/aug/26/parents-children-playtime> (accessed 10 May 2020).

Jung, C. G. (2001) *Modern Man in Search of a Soul.* Oxon: Routledge.

Kaiser Greenland, S. (2016) *Mindful Games.* Boulder, CO: Shambala Publications, Inc.

Kearney, M. (1997) *Mortally Wounded: Stories of Soul, Pain, Death and Healing.* New York: Simon and Schuster.

Keller, J. (2017) *The Psychological Case for Adult Play Time.* Online. HTTP: <https://psmag.com/social-justice/throw-out-your-computer-and-grab-some-legos> (accessed 9 April 2020).

Kidner, C. (2016) *SPICe Briefing: Kinship Care.* Online. HTTP: <www.parliament.scot/ResearchBriefingsAndFactsheets/S5/SB_16-87_Kinship_Care.pdf> (accessed 11 May 2020).

Lachman, M. E. (2015) Mind the gap in the middle: A call to study midlife. *Research in Human Development,* 12 (3–4): 327–334.

Lachman, M. E., Teshale, S. and Agrigoroaei, S. (2015) Midlife as a pivotal period in the life course: Balancing growth and decline at the crossroads of youth and old age. *International Journal of Behavioral Development,* 39: 20–31.

Liberty University (n.d.) *Biosocial Growth in Middle Adulthood.* Online. HTTP: <www.lib erty.edu/courseapps/book/psychology-201/module-7/section-1-title/introduction/> (accessed 30 May 2020).

Ling, Q. (2018) *Forest Bathing: How Trees Can Help You Find Health and Happiness.* New York: Viking.fine.

McManus, S., Bebbington, P., Jenkins, R. and Brugha, T. (Eds.) (2016) *Mental Health and Wellbeing in England: Adult Psychiatric Morbidity Survey 2014.* Leeds: NHS Digital.

Miller, A. L., Rathus, J. H. and Linehan, M. M. (2017) *Dialectical Behaviour Therapy with Suicidal Adolescents.* New York: The Guilford Press.

Mind (2020) *Home.* Online. HTTP: <www.mind.org.uk/> (accessed 13 April 2020).

National Academy for Social Prescribing (2020a) *A Social Revolution in Wellbeing: Strategic Plan 2020–2023.* Online. HTTP: <https://socialprescribingacademy.org.uk/wp-content/uploads/2020/03/NASP_strategic-plan_web.pdf> (accessed 11 September 2020).

National Academy for Social Prescribing (2020b) *Home.* Online. HTTP: <https://socialprescribingacademy.org.uk/> (accessed 11 September 2020).

New Economics Foundation (2011) *Five Ways to Wellbeing: New Applications, New Ways of Thinking.* London: New Economics Foundation.

NHS (2019) *Exercise.* Online. HTTP: <www.nhs.uk/live-well/exercise/#what-counts-as-moderate-aerobic-activity/> (accessed 21 April 2020).

Office for National Statistics (2013) *What Matters Most to Personal Wellbeing.* Online. HTTP: <https://webarchive.nationalarchives.gov.uk/20160107113217/www.ons.gov.uk/ons/rel/wellbeing/measuring-national-well-being/what-matters-most-to-personal-well-being-in-the-uk-/sty-personal-well-being.html> (accessed 16 April 2020).

Office for National Statistics (2019) *Measuring National Well-Being in the UK: International Comparisons, 2019.* Online. HTTP: <www.ons.gov.uk/peoplepopulationandcommunity/wellbeing/articles/measuringnationalwellbeing/internationalcomparisons2019#health> (accessed 16 April 2020).

Pathways Care Farm (2020) *Welcome.* Online. HTTP: <www.pathways-care-farm.org.uk/> (accessed 10 October 2020).

Perry, G. (2014) *Playing to the Gallery.* London: Penguin.

Petelczyc, C. A., Capezio, A., Wang, L. and Restubog, S. L. D. (2018) Play at work: An integrative review and agenda for future research. *Journal of Management,* 44 (1): 161–190.

Phillips, M. L. (2011) *The Mind at Midlife.* Online. HTTP: <www.apa.org/monitor/2011/04/mind-midlife> (accessed 1 June 2020).

Pink, D. H. (2008) *A Whole New Mind: Why Right-Brainers Will Rule the Future.* London: Marshall Cavendish Business.

Pizarro, J. (2004) The efficacy of art and writing therapy: Increasing positive mental health outcomes and participant retention after exposure to traumatic experience. *Art Therapy: Journal of the American Art Therapy Association,* 21 (1): 5–12.

Project Resiliency (2020) *The Benefits of Drumming.* Online. HTTP: <https://project-resiliency.org/resiliency/the-benefits-of-druming/> (accessed 30 May 2020).

Proyer, R. T. (2013) The well-being of playful adults: Adult playfulness, subjective well-being, physical well-being, and the pursuit of enjoyable activities. *European Journal of Humour Research,* 1: 84–98.

Public Health England (2019) *Musculoskeletal Health: Applying All Our Health.* Online. HTTP: <www.gov.uk/government/publications/musculoskeletal-health-applying-all-our-health/musculoskeletal-health-applying-all-our-health> (accessed 12 May 2020).

Public Health England (2020) *Health Matters: Physical Activity – Prevention and Management of Long-Term Conditions.* Online. HTTP: <https://www.gov.uk/government/publications/

health-matters-physical-activity/health-matters-physical-activity-prevention-and-management-of-long-term-conditions> (accessed 17 January 2021).

Raanaas, R. J., Patil, G. G. and Hartig, T. (2011) Health benefits of a view of nature through the window: A quasi-experimental study of patients in a residential rehabilitation center. *Clinical Rehabilitation*, 26 (1): 21–32.

Ratey, J. J. and Hagerman, E. (2010) *Spark! How Exercise Will Improve the Performance of Your Brain*. London: Quercus.

Reuter-Lorenz, P. A. and Park, D. C. (2010) Human neuroscience and the aging mind: A new look at old problems. *The Journals of Gerontology: Series B, Psychological Sciences and Social Sciences*, 65B (4): 405–415.

Rice-Oxley, M. (2019) *Mental Illness: Is There Really a Global Epidemic?* Online. HTTP: <www.theguardian.com/society/2019/jun/03/mental-illness-is-there-really-a-global-epidemic> (accessed 14 April 2020).

Scouts (2020) *Home*. Online. HTTP: <www.scouts.org.uk/> (accessed 21 November 2020).

Sharma, A., Madaan, V. and Petty, F. D. (2006) Exercise for mental health. *Primary Care Companion to Journal of Clinical Psychiatry*, 8 (2): 106.

Sjöberg, B. and Porko-Hudd, M. (2019) A life tangled in yarns: Leisure knitting for well-being. *Techne Series A*, 26 (2): 49–66.

Slawson, N. (2017) *It's Time to Recognise the Contribution Arts Can Make to Health and Wellbeing*. Online. HTTP: <www.theguardian.com/healthcare-network/2017/oct/11/contribution-arts-make-health-wellbeing> (accessed 14 April 2020).

Smith, K. P. and Christakis, N. A. (2008) Social networks and health. *Annual Review of Sociology*, 34: 405–429.

Steel, N., Ford, J., Newton, J., Davis, A., Vos, T., [. . .] and Murray, C. (2018) Changes in health in the countries of the UK and 150 English Local Authority areas 1990–2016: A systematic analysis for the Global Burden of Disease Study 2016. *The Lancet*, 392 (10158): 1647–1661.

Summers, J. K. and Vivian, D. N. (2018) Ecotherapy: A forgotten ecosystem service: A review. *Frontiers in Psychology*, 9: 1389.

Thiel, A., Thedinga, H. K., Thomas, S. L., Barkhoff, H., Giel, K. E., Schweizer, O., Thiel, S. and Zipfe, S. (2016) Have adults lost their sense of play? An observational study of the social dynamics of physical (in)activity in German and Hawaiian leisure settings. *BMC Public Health*, 16 (689): 1–14.

Three Peaks Challenge (2020) *Welcome*. Online. HTTP: <www.threepeakschallenge.uk/> (accessed 21 November 2020).

Tonkin, A. and Whitaker, J. (Eds.) (2016) *Play in Healthcare for Adults: Using Play to Promote Health and Wellbeing throughout the Adult Lifespan*. Oxon: Routledge.

Traynor, M. (2018) Guest editorial: What's wrong with resilience. *Journal of Research in Nursing*, 23 (1): 5–8. doi.org/10.1177/1744987117751458.

Uttley, L., Scope, A., Stevenson, M., [. . .] and Wood, C. (2015) Systematic review and economic modelling of the clinical effectiveness and cost-effectiveness of art therapy among people with non-psychotic mental health disorders. *Health Technology Assessment*, 19 (18): 1–120.

Warburton, A. (2017) *Playmakers*. Online. HTTP: <www.craftscouncil.org.uk/articles/playmakers/> (accessed 10 May 2020).

Whitaker, J. (2019) Finding playfulness in the everyday: An antidote to the 'saturation' of modern family life. In: Tonkin, A. and Whitaker, J. (Eds.), *Play and Playfulness for Public Health and Wellbeing*. Oxon: Routledge: 92–103.

Wilson, J. (2017) *Creativity in Times of Constraint: A Practitioner's Companion in Mental Health and Social Care*. Oxon: Routledge.

Working Families (2019) *Modern Families Index 2019*. Online. HTTP: <https://workingfamilies. org.uk/wp-content/uploads/2019/02/BH_MFI_Report_2019_Full-Report_Final.pdf> (accessed 9 April 2020).

World Health Organization (2020) *The Global Strategy and Action Plan on Ageing and Health*. Online. HTTP: <www.who.int/ageing/global-strategy/en/> (accessed 26 May 2020).

Zak, P. (2011) *Trust, Morality – and Oxytocin*. Online. HTTP: <www.youtube.com/watch? v=rFAdlU2ETjU> (accessed 21 November 2020).

Zimmermann, E. (1971) *Knitting without Tears: Basic Techniques and Easy-to-Follow Directions for Garments to Fit All Sizes*. New York: Charles Scribner's Sons.

8 Elderhood

After decades of hard work in employment, volunteering, child rearing, and caring for parents or older loved ones, the prospect of less responsibility and more time to spend on active leisure seems appealing and just reward for the years of focused activity that make up middle adulthood (Wright 2019). With increasing life expectancy, there is a vested interest in enabling older people to 'age well', so that the knowledge, skills, and experience they have accumulated over many years, might enhance society 'financially, socially and culturally' (Public Health England 2019).

The World Health Organization's (WHO) *Global Healthy Aging Strategy* (Public Health England 2019) identifies 'healthy aging as . . . the process of developing and maintaining the functional ability that enables well-being in older age', promoting the vision that older people will 'have the freedom to be and do what they value'. The notion of personal value is important at this stage of life and can be clearly linked to the last recognized stage of brain maturation. For both men and women, there is a major interest in improving wellbeing and staying healthy (Brizendine 2007, 2011), with factors such as physical and mental abilities and environmental influences all playing their part (Public Health England 2019).

For men, from around the age of 30–40 years, testosterone levels fall by around 2 per cent per year, meaning that by the time they reach the age of 85, their testosterone levels have more than halved in comparison to what they were aged 20 (Brizendine 2011). Lower testosterone levels mark a reduction in aggressiveness and, with lower levels of vasopressin and higher levels of oxytocin now bathing the brain, men become more open to affection as they advance in age. According to Brizendine (2011: 21) 'this is the closest men will ever become to being like women'.

For many women, the menopause is well past, and they enter a postmenopausal equilibrium as low levels of estrogen, testosterone, and lower oxytocin mean that brain circuits are less reactive to stress. Fluctuations in mood subside with the shift in focus from caring for others toward doing what *they* want to do (Brizendine 2007). In John Knight's *Seven Ages of Woman*, this is portrayed as a period of 'freeage after bondage; time – money – freedom – relaxation . . . enjoy, enjoy, enjoy' (Knight 2009).

Morris (2018: 3) states that 'being able to reason, remember, and make decisions the way we always have connects us to the identity, personality traits, and relationships we spend our lives building'. Although the rate of aging is known to accelerate around 65 years of age, how this manifests itself will be dependent upon the decisions made over the course of our lives (Vseteckova 2019). Morris (2018: 10) stresses the importance of reaching elderhood with a well-developed and healthy brain, which 'will have more neurons and neural connections to carry on brain function when neurons die or cell systems fail, both of which are inevitable consequences of aging'.

Adapting to transition and change

Life course theory holds that 'patterns of late-life adaptation and aging are generally linked to the formative years of life course development' (Elder et al. 2003: 11) and Bartlett and Peel (2005: 100) define healthy aging in terms of this capacity for 'adaptation to physical and psychosocial changes across the life course to attain optimal physical, mental and social well being in old-age'. It was Brian Sutton-Smith (1997: 6) who identified the adaptive function of play on account of its 'temporal diversity as well as spatial diversity' and the 'trickle-down' effect by which play skills are transferred to everyday life (*ibid.*: 230). Sutton-Smith argued that play adapts and changes to meet the needs of both players and society, '[allowing] individuals to navigate change, anxiety and sociocultural constraints' (Asbury 2016: 380), while connecting past, present, and future in a meaningful way.

An exploratory study into the meanings attributed to play in later life (Hoppes et al. 2001) found that older adults are motivated to engage in play by their desire for physical and mental fitness; to fill time in a satisfying way; to continue with past hobbies and interests; and to achieve or maintain a sense of belonging. There is now growing evidence to support the view that play contributes to healthy aging by meeting these essential components of physical and mental wellbeing. One example is Yarnal's (2006) study of the *Red Hat Society*, an international organization of women aged over 50, with a mission to 'celebrate the silliness of life'. Yarnal found that membership of this society provided a rule-free context for establishing, nurturing, and maintaining the social relationships upon which healthy aging depends. Further studies found that the benefits of engaging in playful pursuits in a group setting permeate other aspects of life, including relationships with family members (Impact Arts 2011); dealing with day-to-day stresses (Outley and McKenzie 2006); and managing challenging life transitions (Hutchinson et al. 2008).

Mitas et al. (2011) have argued that playfulness could be a crucial component of healthy aging because it allows older people to 'open up' to others, to try new activities, and to cultivate a positive attitude toward growing older. They also hypothesized that playfulness could be both an antecedent of, and component of, the psychological resilience necessary for managing the challenges and changing circumstances associated with aging (*ibid.*). When older adults give themselves permission to play, they are liberated from societal expectations of old age and broaden their repertoire of possibilities, building 'valuable resources including social connections, supportive friendships and dispositional optimism' (*ibid.*: 47).

In the following case-story, Christina Freeman describes how the rediscovery of play helped her to find new meaning in retirement.

Box 8.1 I used to be someone . . . managing the transition to retirement

Christina Freeman

I used to be a healthcare professional with a career of more than 40 years as a clinical diagnostic radiographer, teacher of radiography, and then as a professional lead for education and professional matters. Then I did what the experts say you should never do. I went from a stressful and demanding full-time job to absolutely nothing when I retired. I compounded this by putting my house on the market which rapidly became a replacement activity. We had raised our family in the house, and it was packed full of junk, mementoes of sentimental attachment, and yet more junk. When the house sold, I moved to an area of the country where I knew no one at all.

Little wonder that six months after moving I felt cut adrift and not quite fitting in where I was. I had stayed in contact with good friends and managed to meet them often, but I was missing a community, and home didn't feel like home. I was aware that I needed to take action before I spiraled down to a place where I did not want to be.

A craft and yarn shop in the town offered workshops and I signed up. Daunting as it was to be surrounded by talented craftspeople, there was something soothing in the rhythmic jabbing of needle-felting and joy to be had in producing something, albeit slightly wonky. Knitting was next on the list and I found that, as long as I stuck to knitting squares or triangles, this too was a relaxing process. I felt soothed and it occurred to me that I had, in effect, rediscovered the joy of simply mucking about. As a working professional (coupled with bringing up children, keeping house, looking after husband), I had lost sight of the joy of simply *being* rather than rushing around *doing*.

Spurred-on with a little more confidence, I undertook a six-week course at a local pottery center. I thought I would be good at it but, by the end of the course, I had not produced anything remotely worth taking home. At this stage I might have given up but, having rediscovered the possibility of fun, I wasn't ready to throw in the towel. I registered as a member of the center, which allows me to go to the pottery studio one day a week. I love my Wednesdays there; I take a packed lunch and spend the day just fiddling around. It has given me a renewed sense of calm and I am able to laugh at my efforts. It doesn't matter that I'm not the best potter in the world, I still experience a sense of joy. I don't have to produce beautiful pots; if that's what I wanted, I could go out and buy them. What I want is time when my brain is focused on something that doesn't actually matter. I find that the repetitive movements involved in pottery making free the brain to do something else at the same time.

I am now happy and settled in my forever home. I go to a Pilates class which, although more work than fun, at least keeps me active. I have local friends and acquaintances who I have met through my various activities. My mental health is strong, and my physical health is way better than it was when I was working. I have realized something very important – that I don't have to be successful or to prove anything to anyone. I am free just to play and to enjoy my life.

Throughout our lives, the brain changes more than any other part of the body and, as with all other body systems, increasing age sees a natural decline in brain function (Nichols 2017). The older brain is characterized by cognitive decline which manifests in altered functionality: 'our ability to think slows down, and we may experience occasional difficulty in, for example, recalling where we left our keys or retrieving a word or name. By all accounts, this is considered a normal degree of cognitive decline' (Morris 2018 Kindle Loc 81).

Emerging research has identified a link between retirement and a decline in cognitive functioning (Wright 2019). Speed of processing is indicative of a healthy brain network, and a decline in processing speed is recognized as a main indicator of brain aging; when it takes longer to process information, there is an increased likelihood of forgetfulness and confusion (*ibid.*). It has been suggested that, in retirement, alternative sources of intellectual stimulation may be needed to substitute for work-related mental activity (Andel, cited in Wright 2019).

For people who work long hours for many years, there may be limited opportunities to pursue personal interests and hobbies and when it is time to retire, surplus time and how to fill it can become a source of concern (Age UK 2020). One of the *Five Ways to Wellbeing* (New Economics Foundation 2020) is to '*Give*' and one of the suggested ways of 'giving' is to 'volunteer your time'. This is particularly beneficial to the older individual when it is linked to the wider community because, as well as meeting the needs of the recipients of voluntary endeavor, it can also 'be incredibly rewarding and [create] connections with the people around you' (*ibid.*). The following case-story from Irene Lawrence shows how volunteering can lead to unexpectedly playful benefits when the volunteer community comes together.

Box 8.2 Nerf guns and ripped T-shirts: volunteers at play

Irene Lawrence

Church volunteers were invited to an evening of treats – food and drink, games (with prizes!) – as a thank you for participating in community events. We were a mixed age group, mainly youth workers and a few of us older people with time on our hands.

I was excited when I realized the variety of games on offer, although I found out very quickly that I was not as hot at table football as I thought I was – youth workers often played in their lunch breaks while I was out of practice. However, a Nerf gun challenge was right up my street; I felt more confident at this as I have an eye for distance and aim. I won the prize for 'best shot' and declined to reveal that archery was my main hobby, in which I regularly compete!

There were various quizzes and brain games available, but these didn't really interest me as I was now too excited by other physical and aiming challenges.

The last game of the evening was a mystery – details of which were not divulged prior to the start. We were asked to split into two teams, with one person from each team blindfolded. The remainder of the team then had to shout out instructions for navigating an obstacle course across the large church hall, through a door and into a smaller adjoining room where the blindfolded player had to grab a stuffed toy. As the game commenced and I was blindfolded, I quickly realized that being hearing impaired I wasn't receiving clear instructions. Surrounded by the loud shouts from each team, which echoed around the hall, I began to feel a sense of rising panic as I was left standing while the other team gained headway. I became aware that someone was shouting, 'she can't hear you, she can't hear anything', prompting one member of my team to come closer to me. I was able to continue the game and quickly caught up, reaching the end of the course at the same time as my male counterpart. Relief, panic, and my competitive spirit spurred me on to make a grab for the target. Determined not to fail at the last hurdle, I tugged and tugged at the 'stuffed toy', not realizing that what I had hold of was in fact my opponent's T-shirt, which I almost ripped in my eagerness to win. Much embarrassment and laughter followed – but I did recompense the loser for the price of his shirt!

On reflection, part of the fun in being older is that you can be a little less inhibited about play. Best of all, you might look older, but don't feel it; you can continue to surprise yourself and others. The downside is that not everyone remembers to play as they get older. In the words of George Bernard Shaw, 'We don't stop playing because we grow old; we grow old because we stop playing'.

Play: a ticket out of loneliness

As outlined in the Introduction to this book, these chapters were penned during the onset of the global pandemic of 2020. The restrictions on movement and social interaction which characterized governmental responses to the crisis exposed whole populations to the concept of 'social isolation', as we collectively withdrew from everyday social activities to 'lock-down' in our own homes. For many this was the first experience of real loneliness, and the associated rise in physical and mental health problems unrelated to the coronavirus (e.g., Health & Equity in Recovery Plans Working Group 2020; Regan and Chi 2020) underlined what was already a growing concern about the impact of loneliness – especially among older people. At a time when human sociality was challenged by restrictive public health directives, the adaptive benefits of play and playfulness were revealed in a myriad of community initiatives designed to counter the repercussions of social isolation (Tonkin and Whitaker 2020).

With the advancing years, many people spend more time alone than when they were younger, making them more vulnerable to social isolation and loneliness. The term 'social isolation' defines the objective state of physical separation from other people, while 'loneliness' is the subjective experience of distress associated with being alone or separated from others, whether physically or emotionally (National Institute on Aging 2019). In the UK, over half of all people aged over 75 live on their own (Office for National Statistics 2017), and half a million older people can go several days without seeing another person (Mortimer 2016). This compares with an estimated 28 per cent of older adults who live on their own in the US (US Department of Health and Human Services 2018). Age UK predicts that, by 2025–2026, the number of people experiencing loneliness after middle age is set to reach two million, a 49 per cent increase over the course of ten years (Age UK 2018).

Loneliness is regarded as one of the greatest health risks for older adults, increasing the likelihood of premature death by 29 per cent (Holt-Lunstad et al. 2015). Living alone, poor social connections, and loneliness have been found to pose the equivalent health risk to smoking 15 cigarettes per day (Holt-Lunstad et al. 2010) and to be more damaging to health than obesity (*ibid.*). Various studies have found that lonely people are more likely to suffer from depression (Cacioppo et al. 2006); cognitive decline (James et al. 2011); heart disease, and stroke (Valtorta et al. 2016) than the general population – with obvious implications for quality of life in elderhood.

Age UK have been at the forefront of research into different approaches to tackling the problem of loneliness in later life. They have found that the most 'promising approaches' (Jopling 2015) are not specific activities or interventions, but rather services which address one or more of the key challenges faced in working with lonely individuals. These are identified as: *reaching* lonely individuals; *understanding* and responding to their unique set of circumstances; and *supporting* individuals to engage with services which could lead to meaningful social connections (*ibid.*: 12). Experts agree that the problems associated with loneliness do not demand specific 'loneliness solutions' but 'holistic and person-centered services, aimed at promoting healthy and active ageing, building resilience, and supporting independence' (*ibid*.: 12). It is evident that the best way to tackle the problem of loneliness among older adults is to take a preventive stance, which promotes the independence and autonomy of older individuals, averts deterioration in their physical or mental wellbeing, and so delays the need for more intensive – and costly – intervention (Windle et al. 2011).

Examples of best practice cited by Age UK (2018) center around relationships – reviving and maintaining existing relationships; building new connections; and promoting positive mental health. Central to these research findings, and the recommendations that follow from them, is the importance of recognizing each person as an individual, with unique challenges, strengths, and interests, which can provide starting points for support (National Institute of Health and Care Excellence [NICE] 2012). Everyone experiences aging in a unique and individual way which is influenced by their personal history and by the sociocultural context of their past and present lives, factors which also influence the rate of cognitive decline (Morris 2018). Age UK (2018) recognizes the need for creativity and imagination in designing person-centered services which are empowering to the older individual, while also addressing societal constraints to personal autonomy and choice.

Age UK research into wellbeing in later life (Green et al. 2017) found that engagement in creative and cultural activities makes the greatest contribution to general wellbeing in later life and a report by the All Party Parliamentary Group (APPG) on Arts, Health and Wellbeing (2017) offers snapshots of how arts organizations contribute to healthy aging through dance, music, singing, the written and spoken word, and the creative and performing arts. The report presents a comprehensive bank of evidence for the fiscal benefits of prevention linked to healthy aging, including falls prevention, combating social isolation, and delaying the onset of dementia, reinforcing the proposition that 'arts engagement may lead to longer lives better lived' (APPG on Arts, Health and Wellbeing: 122).

The following case-story describes an initiative in Scotland that highlights the drive for play which underlies the creative impulse and which connects us to our inner selves, to each other, and to our physical and social environment.

Box 8.3 Everyday magic. Celebrating choice and self-expression at Impact Arts' Craft Café

Impact Arts, established in 1994, is a forward-thinking community arts organization which uses creativity and the arts to enable and empower social change. Working collaboratively with children, young people, older adults, and communities, Impact Arts places innovation, enterprise, and creativity alongside outstanding delivery, sound management, and a strong ethos of partnership to tackle society's big issues.

Craft Café is Impact Art's flagship program for older people. It offers a safe, social, and creative environment in which older people can learn new skills, renew social networks, and reconnect with the local community. Craft Café has two distinct models of delivery, one within a community setting, the second within a care home; the principles of self-directed learning and choice flow through both models, as does the aim to connect with the wider community.

Craft Café offers morning and afternoon sessions four days a week. Participants, who range in age from 60 to 101, are welcomed with refreshments and given time to settle in and catch up with friends before embarking on their own individual projects or engaging with a group theme (Figure 8.1). Previous themes have included everything from Chinese New Year, International Women's Day, art movements, botanical illustration, stories and myths, to recycling and creative ecology. Group members can choose from a wide variety of artistic media, from drawing to painting, sculpture to craft work, reading to storytelling, with artists in residence acting as teachers and facilitators who guide and support each member on their creative journey. The warm welcome and set-up of the sessions creates a safe space within which participants can try out new things in a supportive social context, while offering structure to those who need it.

Karen discovered Craft Café two years ago, while visiting a friend in her care home. She was accompanied by Breck, her friend's 14-year-old border terrier, which has also become a regular and popular guest at the Craft Café. Karen had not done any form of artistic activity for 50 years, since being told in primary school that she would never be able to draw or paint, but with gentle encouragement she began by coloring mandalas, before going on to create her own intricate designs which were then transferred to a set of ceramic tiles. The Craft Café unleashed Karen's latent creative potential and she has grown in confidence to take on increasingly bold artistic challenges, while enlivening the group with her positive, cheerful energy.

Craft Café is a creative innovation which has had a positive impact on many people's lives (Impact Arts 2011). It provides a stimulating, engaging, yet peaceful space where members can spend time, socialize, explore their creativity, and express themselves. The element of choice is at the heart of Craft Cafe: participants choose whether and when to engage with the art and are free to decide what to do – even if that is just to stop by for coffee. Through these principles of freedom and choice, members retain ownership of the space which allows for an 'opening-up' to the creative possibilities of playful exploration.

Play is at the heart of everything that Craft Cafe represents. Intrinsically motivated engagement harnesses the joy of creativity, artistic expression, and learning, and from this arise playfulness, spontaneity, and fun. In the words of Karen, this is 'something which should be experienced by so many people regardless of who they are, what stage they are in life and whether they have artistic talent or not'.

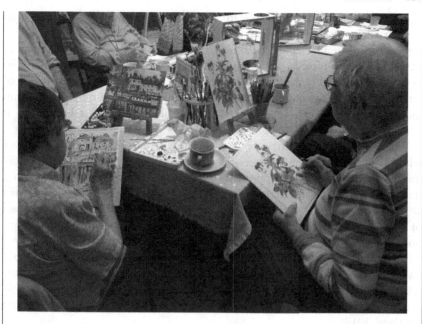

Figure 8.1 Impact Arts, Craft Café

Source: Photograph by Rachel McEwen.

The *Five Pillars of Aging Well* are nutrition, hydration, physical, social, and cognitive stimulation (Vseteckova 2019), which can be redefined as 'exercising, learning new tasks, keeping socially active . . . [and having] the right foods to fuel the brain' (Morris 2018). In 2008, as part of the UK Government's Foresight Project, Haworth and Roberts (2008) were commissioned to explore the importance of leisure for mental capital and wellbeing. Promoting the role of *active leisure* (both physical and non-physical) as a means of reducing depression and anxiety, producing positive moods, and enhancing psychological wellbeing, Haworth and Roberts (2008: 4) declared that 'maintaining motivation for active leisure is only possible if it is marked by enjoyment'. The contribution exercise makes to a better functioning brain cannot be understated (Morris 2018), and here the contribution of play comes to the fore.

Finding the fun in fitness

Older adults are among the least active members of society (Australian Institute for Health and Welfare 2017), yet even a small increase in physical activity can significantly improve health and wellbeing across physiological, psychological, and social dimensions. Research reveals marked health benefits even among those who take up some form of physical activity for the first time in their later years (Hamer et al. 2014). A review of older people's participation in sport (Stenner et al. 2019) identifies factors related to community and friendship as key motivators for continued participation in sporting activities in later life and, in contrast to the popular view of people slowing down or 'mellowing' with age, Stenner et al. (*ibid.*) found competition to be another motivating factor, expressed in a desire for challenge and the achievement of personal goals.

Rigby (2013) recalls the tale of Ken, an 85-year-old table tennis player who challenged a much younger player to 'put money on it' – before duly trashing his unsuspecting opponent. This anecdote contrasts starkly with a statement by author and lifelong ping-pong player, Pico Iyer (cited in Adrian 2019), who says that 'In Japan, a game of ping-pong is really like an act of love – you're taught to play with somebody, rather than against somebody'. Research suggests that ping-pong may be helpful to older people with dementia (Adrian 2019) because it 'combines physical activity with spatial skills, cognition and keeping social' (Rigby 2013). It seems likely that, whether played competitively or just for fun, 'the combination of gentle exercise and plenty of socializing [creates] the perfect mix' (Open Access Scotland 2017).

Physical activity can take many forms besides sport or formal exercise, including walking (to the shops or in nature), gardening, dancing, and playing with grandchildren or pets – all of which may incorporate features of play and the playful: intrinsic motivation, imagination, and subjective wellbeing.

Research into the health benefits of dance, for example, shows that it increases people's motivation to engage in sustained physical activity because dance is perceived as fun, expressive, sociable, and non-competitive (Department of Health 2011). The Royal Academy of Dance's *Silver Swans* ballet program (Royal Academy of Dance 2020) is especially designed for older dancers and aims to improve mobility, posture, coordination, and energy in the context of a supportive social group. By way of contrast, the 2014 documentary film Hiphop-eration (Hiphop-eration n.d.) describes the formation of a Hip-Hop dance troupe in New Zealand, with an average age of nearly 80! Significantly, dance fosters positive social interaction and encourages participation in new physical, social, and recreational activities, creating a positive upward spiral of lifestyle changes and a bank of enduring and transferable personal resources (Fredrickson and Joiner 2018).

In Scotland, Scottish Ballet (2020) currently runs three Dance Health programs which have reached more than 1,000 participants since the project's inception in 2015. *Time to Dance* is designed for people living with dementia and their carers, while *Elevate©* aims to improve the physical, mental, and social wellbeing of people living with multiple sclerosis. The following case-story offers an insight into Scottish Ballet's third groundbreaking program, Dance for Parkinson's *Scotland*, delivered in partnership with Dance Base (n.d.), which uncovers the 'play' within the dance.

Box 8.4 'It's like being given permission to be free': the role of 'play' within Dance for Parkinson's Scotland

Bethany Whiteside and Lisa Sinclair

'The strains of Løvenskjold's score rippled across the room as we all scrunched up our bodies and faces and then slowly opened them up to reveal the particular emotion, *mischievous*, called for by Miriam. We widened our eyes, gave pert little smiles, and drummed our fingers against our lips. Two of the dancers stuck their tongues out at each other and then convulsed in laughter. Scottish Ballet's current repertoire is Matthew Bourne's 'Highland Fling' and, we too, are being Sylphs. Childish, playful creatures who danced the emotions that they felt' (Field notes recorded at Scottish Ballet, April 2017, by Bethany Whiteside).

Dance for Health is a rapidly evolving field of practice and study situated within, and across, the academic, arts, health, and social care sectors. Shaping its narrative is the global phenomenon that is the Dance for Parkinson's movement, spanning numerous classes, companies, and countries. The core premise is simple: the practice is dance and dancer-centered and works with the 'whole' dancer through meeting individual cultural, social, emotional, and physical needs.

'Dance structures, such as movement tasks and improvisation scores, which demand cooperation amongst dancers, lead to play' (Houston 2019: 136). The aforementioned extract from field notes demonstrates the power of guided creative movement to spontaneously lead to a moment of shared joy.

Playfulness and humor are core and constant threads embedded within the Dance for Parkinson's Scotland (DfPS) program (Figure 8.2) run in partnership by Scottish Ballet and Dance Base, Edinburgh and enabled and encouraged in interlinked ways. Through, for example: exploiting the spontaneity inherent to creative movement; enabling dancers to take ownership of their situation through humor; having a specific focus on exploration of emotions; the ability of the live musicians to create and respond 'in the moment'; learning and drawing on individual and collective personalities and narratives; and, lastly, recognizing generational needs and experiences. Focusing on just the latter aspect here, dancers convey the value of the play experience for them: 'I feel like a child again. I can be silly again' (Interview with dancer at Scottish Ballet, Whiteside 2017).

'We're of the generation where my grandparents were still Edwardians and they believed that children should be seen and not heard, so you didn't express yourself at home, you sat there a lot of the time and behaved and it's taken a long time to shed that . . . And I think, suddenly *it's like being given permission to be free*' (interview with dancer at Dance Base, Whiteside 2017, emphasis added).

The value of experiencing 'fun' through participation is receiving increased attention (see, e.g. Houston 2019) counteracting a dominance within research to focus on the physical impact of dancing for people with Parkinson's. Simply put, the practice enables each dancer to have 'the jester's licence to broaden [their] horizon' (Klausmann 2015 in Houston 2019: 142). Certainly, the DfPS dancers and practitioners embrace and use this 'licence' in a creative myriad of wonderful ways.

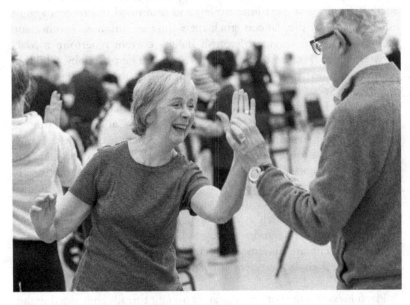

Figure 8.2 Playfulness and humor are embedded in the Dance for Parkinson's Scotland program

Source: Photograph by Andy Ross Images.

The rhythm of the gardening year is an apt metaphor for growth throughout the lifespan: seeds sown in childhood and nurtured through the teenage years, come into fruit in midlife and by elderhood, they are ready for harvest. There is a growing body of evidence supporting the benefits of community growing for physical and mental wellbeing, including for older people. An example is the Growing Well project (Federation of City Farms and Community Gardens 2018), which highlights the effectiveness of therapeutic gardening in tackling the loneliness and social isolation often experienced by older people, including those with dementia, combining meaningful physical activity with exposure to nature in a communal setting. In a review of the relevant literature, Wright and Wadsworth (2014) conclude that gardening impacts on the health of older people in specific ways, but 'there is the added dimension of what the garden symbolizes psychologically as a meaningful reason for existence, or as one older adult expressed it, "when I'm in the garden I can create my own paradise"' (*ibid.* 8).

Another motivator for physical activity is pet ownership (Knight and Edwards 2008). Studies have found an association between owning a pet and increased physical activity in older adults (e.g., Curl et al. 2017). Knight and Edwards (2008) found that older people feel safer walking when accompanied by a dog, which also creates opportunities for building and maintaining social relationships. Wood et al. (2015) report that 40 per cent of pet owners surveyed, received tangible support from people they met through their animal companions.

Creating a playful landscape

With many people living longer, healthier lives (World Health Organization 2020), there is an increasing realization that older adults 'can be creative, productive, carers, lovers, citizens, consumers and enjoyers of what society has to offer' (Marmot 2015: 203). However, it remains the case that a medley of individual, social, and environmental factors combine to influence participation in physical and social activity by older adults, who may face complex personal and environmental barriers to becoming and remaining active (British Heart Foundation National Centre for Physical Activity and Health 2012). An increasing range of creative initiatives has been specifically designed with the aim of improving accessibility for those living with age-related disabilities or health conditions, or in adverse social circumstances – many of which revolve around a playful core (APPG on Arts, Health and Wellbeing 2017).

While the majority of older people continue to live in their own homes, 4 per cent of those over 65 and 15 per cent of those aged over 85 live in residential care facilities and 40 per cent of care home residents require specialist dementia care (MHA 2020). The College of Occupational Therapists (2015) has developed a toolkit entitled *Living well through activity in care homes*, which promotes active engagement through familiar sources of enjoyment based on the individual's personal history. While this initiative emphasizes self-care and personal leisure, one of three cited contributors to a good home life is *connecting*. According to the APPG on Arts, Health and Wellbeing (2017: 130) 'arts participation in care homes helps to safeguard mental health, wellbeing and independence in older people'.

Listening to music, making music, and dance are integral to the lives of all of us, and recent research by Philip et al. (2019) supports the view that such everyday pastimes may have additional benefits for those living with chronic illness or infirmity. The health benefits of singing, for example, include the need to focus attention and control breathing, offering protection against stress and anxiety while 'raising the spirits and making people happy' (APPG on Arts, Health and Wellbeing 2017: 123). *Singing for Lung Health* is an example of a group-based arts in health intervention which aims to improve the quality of life of people with chronic lung conditions, as well as providing tools for the self-management of breathlessness (British Lung Foundation (BLF) 2020). John (cited in BLF 2020) describes the playful engagement at the heart of the singing sessions: 'We start with some breathing and singing exercises. Some of these involve making funny faces and funny noises – we always have a good laugh'. By helping participants to manage the symptoms of breathlessness, group singing can lead to improved quality of life, mood, activities of daily living, and participation in meaningful social and physical activity (The Musical Breath 2020).

Silver Songs Clubs (APPG on Arts, Health and Wellbeing 2017: 123) promote community singing with the slogan 'A song a day keeps the doctor away' and in the following case-story, deputy care home manager, Jo Vigar, explains her decision to introduce more opportunities for communal singing for her residents.

Box 8.5 Singing together – our dementia choir

Jo Vigar

Working in a residential care home, I have often noticed how music benefits our residents, especially residents with dementia. It can help reduce anxiety and depression, maintain speech and language, and generally enhances the quality of life and atmosphere in the home. Everyone remembers songs from the past: their first kiss, a song at their wedding, watching their parents dance; and we often use music to remember people at funerals. I have noticed how music lights up emotional memories in our residents and, toward the end of life, music and memory can create a powerful connection.

We have always encouraged our residents to sing and when I watched a television documentary in May 2019 called *Our Dementia Choir* (BBC 2021), I felt a real empathy with the singers' enjoyment, happiness, and sense of purpose and I decided that the residents in my care home could really benefit from communal singing. I decided to advertise for someone to come to the home to have a singalong with the residents, to music from their era. I hoped this would promote a connection with the music they listened to in their younger days as this can bring back fond memories. I was hoping that *our* version of a dementia choir would also stimulate levels of engagement – if even just for an hour or so.

We were fortunate to have a volunteer reply to our advert and, every other week, they would come in to engage with a small group of residents. Watching how the residents responded to the opportunity for communal singing was really interesting, because it did not always lead to the anticipated outcomes. There were distinctly different responses from three of our residents and, when we explored their backgrounds, we discovered that music had been an integral part of their earlier lives.

One resident became very tearful as soon as the choir started. She didn't really join in the singing but would interact by dancing along to the music. Now, when we find her tearful, we put on some music and this changes her mood instantly and she will stand up and start to dance. Another resident with advanced dementia had been unable to speak for quite a few months. When the choir was performing, she moved her lips as though singing along, miming the words, tapping her feet, and smiling with her eyes. We know that this lady loved music, singing, and dancing in her early days, and when the singing stopped you could see by her facial expressions that she still enjoys it; the smile remained on her face for the rest of the day. A third resident, who used to sing and play the piano when she was younger, and who always seems to enjoy listening to music, did not like the choir at all. She complained that the choir 'made a racket', causing unnecessary noise and asked to be removed from the room until the choir practice had finished.

Listening to and engaging with music is a universal experience; it reflects and directs our mood and stays with us throughout our lives. However, the reactions of our residents are a reminder that how we respond to music may change over time and communal singing can impact us in a variety of ways that go beyond the actual experience.

Embracing digital play

Since its creation 30 years ago, the internet has become the primary source of information, services, and interpersonal connection for most people, and it has an important role to play in helping older adults maintain their independence and social connections. There are now more people online in later life than ever before, and in recent years the proportion of older adults using the internet has risen faster than for the general population (Richardson 2018). However, this belies the fact that older people are more likely not to have used the internet at all: in 2017, the over 55s made up 78 per cent of those who have never been online, and those over 75, more than half of non-users (*ibid.*). This has led to a debate about the impact of digital technology on the health and wellbeing of older adults (Campaign to End Loneliness 2020). Some argue that the global predominance of digital communication has exacerbated the exclusion of older people (e.g., Campbell 2008), while others identify its potential for enabling older people to maintain and expand their social connections (Ayres 2012).

Previous discussion has emphasized social connection as a central component of health and wellbeing in later life and the internet offers new possibilities for socialization among older internet users (Leist 2013). In a study of the 'fun culture' in the online social networks of older adults, Nimrod (2010) identifies the playful nature of their online communications. This is evident in their creative play, joking, and sociable conversation and suggests 'a sense of regeneration and recreation' (*ibid.*: 234). Nimrod concluded that the 'unique features' of the fun culture characteristic of older people's online communities 'enable[s] meaningful play, liminality, and communitas' (*ibid.*: 235), and its positive impact on the daily lives of participants may be because it encourages social and mental engagement, which are themselves key aspects of healthy aging.

Digital gaming has become an engaging and enjoyable pastime for many older people. It draws them into a world of play: 'fictitious, puzzling, fantasy, and educational situations where they must meet challenges, compete, and win rewards' (Kaufman et al. (2020: 6). Recent research by the American Association of Retired Persons (AARP) (Nelson-Kakulla 2020) found that 44 per cent of older Americans play video games as a form of relaxation and that over half of these feel that online gaming has a positive impact on their wellbeing (*ibid.*). The mastery of new skills, and the setting and achievement of personal goals, allows the player to enter a state of 'flow', a play zone distinct from day-to-day life (Csikszentmihalyi 1997).

Kaufman et al. (2020) find that playing digital games can support and extend other measures for meeting the previously described challenges associated with aging. 'Exergames', for example, which encourage older adults to be more active by combining movement with game features have been linked to improvement in specific physical functions, including balance, mobility, strength, flexibility, function after knee replacement, and walking speed and endurance (Chao et al. 2015).

Digital gaming has also been shown to enhance older adults' cognitive function (Zhang and Kaufman 2016). The AARP reports that the most popular digital games among older people are puzzle and logic games (50 per cent), card and tile games (48 per cent), and trivia, word, and video board games (24 per cent), and that the majority (85 per cent) of older adults who play video games also play traditional versions of the same games (Nelson-Kakulla 2020). A study by Altschul and Deary (2020) found that playing these traditional games is linked to a reduced decline in thinking skills, particularly memory and thinking speed, and similar findings arise from studies into the cognitive impact of digital gaming (e.g., Kaufman et al. 2018).

Neurological research has established the role of the hippocampus in maintaining cognitive function: several studies suggest that stimulation of the hippocampus increases both functional activity and gray matter within this region (e.g., West et al. 2017). It may be that playing video games can trigger this reaction in older people, with implications for preventing and treating cognitive decline in later life. Scientists from across traditional academic divisions are increasingly inspired to work collaboratively to tackle the challenges posed by an aging population with the potential for more people to reach elderhood as healthier and more active individuals.

Conclusion

The College of Occupational Therapists neatly encapsulates older age stating: 'Getting older is not a disease or a condition; and although old age often involves loss, we do not lose the ability to make choices, learn or experience love and affection' (College of Occupational Therapists (2015: 1). In the twenty-first century, elderhood is being reconceptualized as a time of opportunity, when time and energy are no longer dedicated to work or to raising a family. Societal acceptance that older people can continue to participate and contribute as active citizens opens the door to playful endeavor in all its guises.

References

Adrian, J. (2019) *Life Lessons from Ping Pong*. Online. HTTP: <https://medium.com/@jonathanoei/ping-pong-8342d3b3cc22> (accessed 20 September 2020).

Age UK (2018) *All the Lonely People: Loneliness in Later Life*. Online. HTTP: <www.ageuk.org.uk/globalassets/age-uk/documents/reports-and-publications/reports-and-briefings/loneliness/loneliness-report.pdf> (accessed 11 May 2020).

Age UK (2020) *Preparing Emotionally for Retirement*. Online. HTTP: <www.ageuk.org.uk/information-advice/work-learning/retirement/preparing-emotionally-for-retirement/> (accessed 26 May 2020).

All Party Parliamentary Group on Arts, Health and Wellbeing (2017) Online. HTTP: <www.culturehealthandwellbeing.org.uk/appg-inquiry/> (accessed 14 April 2020).

Altschul, D. R. and Deary, I. J. (2020) Playing analog games is associated with reduced declines in cognitive function: A 68-year longitudinal cohort study. *The Journals of Gerontology: Series B*, 75 (3): 474–482.

Asbury, S. (2016) Serious fun: A 'strong' model for play and folklore in children's museums. In: Dewhurst, C. K., Hall, P. and Seemann, C. (Eds.), *Folklife and Museums: Twenty-First Century Perspectives*. Lanham, MD: Rowman and Littlefield.

Australian Institute for Health and Welfare (2017) *Insufficient Physical Activity*. Online. HTTP: <www.aihw.gov.au/reports/risk-factors/risk-factors-to-health/contents/insufficient-physical-activity> (accessed 12 may 2020).

Ayres, S. (2012) *How the Internet and Digital Technology Can Combat Isolation*. Online. HTTP: <How the internet and digital technology can combat isolation> (accessed 21 May 2020).

Bartlett, H. and Peel, N. (2005) Healthy ageing in the community. In: Andrews, G.J. and Phillips, D. R. (Eds.), *Ageing and Place: Perspectives, Policy and Practice*. New York: Routledge.

BBC (2021) *Our Dementia Choir with Vicky McClure*. Online. HTTP: <https://www.bbc.co.uk/programmes/m0004pyg> (accessed 13 January 2021).

British Heart Foundation National Centre for Physical Activity and Health (2012) *Physical Activity for Older Adults: Evidence Briefing*. Online. HTTP: <www.ncsem-em.org.uk/wp-content/uploads/2018/11/older_adults_evidence_briefing.pdf> (accessed 14 May 2020).

British Lung Foundation (2020) *Singing for Lung Health*. Online. HTTP: <www.blf.org.uk/support-for-you/singing-for-lung-health> (accessed 14 August 2020).

Brizendine, L. (2007) *The Female Brain*. New York: Bantam Books.

Brizendine, L. (2011) *The Male Brain: An Essential Owner's Manual for Every Man, and a Cheat Sheet for Every Woman*. New York: Bantam Books.

Cacioppo, J. T., Hughes, M. E., Waite, L. J., Hawkley, L. C. and Thisted, R. A. (2006) Loneliness as a specific risk factor for depressive symptoms: Cross-sectional and longitudinal analyses. *Psychology and Aging*, 21 (1): 140–151.

Campaign to End Loneliness (2020) *Technology: Will It Ever Be a 'Fix' for Loneliness?* Online. HTTP: <www.campaigntoendloneliness.org/blog/technology-loneliness-fix/> (accessed 21 May 2020).

Campbell, A. (2008) Internet use and loneliness in older adults. *Cyberpsychology and Behavior*, 1 (2): 208–211.

Chao, Y.-Y., Scherer, Y. K. and Montgomery, C. A. (2015) Effects of using Nintendo Wii™ exergames in older adults: A review of the literature. *Journal of Aging and Health*, 27 (3): 379–402.

College of Occupational Therapists (2015) *Living Well through Activity in Care Homes: The Toolkit*. London: College of Occupational Therapists.

Csikszentmihalyi, M. (1997) Flow and education. *NAMTA Journal*, 22 (2): 2–35.

Curl, A. L., Bibbo, J. and Johnson, R. A. (2017) Dog walking, the human-animal bond and older adults' physical health. *Gerontologist*, 57: 930–939.

Dance Base (n.d.) *Home*. Online. HTTP: <www.dancebase.co.uk/> (accessed 28 May 2020).

Department of Health (2011) *Cool Facts, Hot Feet: Dancing to Health: A Review of the Evidence*. Online. HTTP: <www.communitydance.org.uk/DB/resources-3/cool-facts-hot-feet-dancing-to-health-a-review-of-> (accessed 14 May 2020).

Elder, G., Johnson, M. and Crosnoe, R. (2003) The emergence and development of life course theory. In: Mortimer, J. and Shanahan, M. (Eds.), *Handbook of the Life Course: Handbooks of Sociology and Social Research*. Boston, MA: Springer.

Federation of City Farms and Community Gardens (2018) *Benefits of Community Growing: Older People and Dementia Sufferers*. Online. HTTP: www.farmgarden.org.uk/sites/farmgarden.org.uk/files/benefits-community-growing-older-people-dementia.pdf (accessed 14 May 2020).

Fredrickson, B. L. and Joiner, T. (2018) Reflections on positive emotions and upward spirals. *Perspectives in Psychological Science*, 13 (2): 194–199.

Green, M., Iparraguirre, J., Davidson, S., Rossall, P. and Zaidi, A. (2017) *A Summary of Age UK's Index of Wellbeing in Later Life*. London: Age UK.

Hamer, L., Lavoie, K. L. and Bacon, S. L. (2014) Taking up physical activity in later life and healthy ageing: The English longitudinal study of ageing. *British Journal of Sports Medicine*, 48 (3): 239–243.

Haworth, J. and Roberts, K. (2008) *State-of-Science Review: SR-C8 Leisure: The Next 25 Years*. London: The Government Office for Science.

Health & Equity in Recovery Plans Working Group (2020) *Direct and Indirect Impacts of COVID-19 on Health and Wellbeing*. Online. HTTP: <www.ljmu.ac.uk/~/media/phi-reports/2020-07-direct-and-indirect-impacts-of-covid19-on-health-and-wellbeing.pdf> (accessed 22 September 2020).

Hiphop-eration (n.d.) *Home*. Online. HTTP: <https://hiphoperationthemovie.com/> (accessed 14 May 2020).

Holt-Lunstad, J., Smith, T. B., Baker, M., Harris, T. and Stephenson, D. (2015) Loneliness and social isolation as risk factors for mortality: A meta-analytic review. *Perspectives on Psychological Science*, 10 (2): 227–237.

Holt-Lunstad, J., Smith, T. B. and Layton, J. B. (2010) Social relationships and mortality risk: A meta-analytic review. *PLoS Medicine*, 7 (7): e1000316.

Hoppes, S., Wilcox, T. and Graham, G. (2001) Meanings of play for older adults. *Physical and Occupational Therapy in Geriatrics*, 18: 57–68.

Houston, S. (2019) *Dancing with Parkinson's*. Bristol, UK: Intellect.

Hutchinson, S. L., Yarnal, C., Son, J. and Kerstetter, D. (2008) Beyond fun and friendship: The Red Hat Society® as a coping resource for older women. *Ageing and Society*, 28: 979–999.

Impact Arts (2011) *Craft Café: Creative Solutions to Isolation and Loneliness: Social Return on Investment Evaluation*. Online. HTTP: <www.impactarts.co.uk/content/about-publica tions/Craft-Cafe-SROI-Summary.pdf> (accessed 18 May 2020).

James, B. D., Wilson, R. S., Barnes, L. L. and Bennett, D. A. (2011) Late-life social activity and cognitive decline in old age. *Journal of the International Neuropsychological Society*, 17 (6): 998-1005.

Jopling, K. (2015) *Promising Approaches to Reducing Loneliness and Isolation in Later Life*. London: Age UK.

Kaufman, D., Gayowsky, T., Sauvé, L., Renaud, L. and Duplàa, E. (2018) Benefits of digital games for older adults: Associations with demographics and game use patterns. *Gerontechnology*, 17 (1): 57–68.

Kaufman, D., Sauve, L. and Ireland, A. (2020) *Playful Aging: Digital Games for Older Adults*. A White Paper by the AGE-WELL 4.2 Project. Online. HTTP: <https://agewell-nce.ca/wp-content/uploads/2020/02/AGE-WELL_WP4.2_White-paper_GAMES.pdf> (accessed 20 May 2020).

Knight, J. (2009) *Seven Ages of Woman*. Online. HTTP: <www.poemhunter.com/poem/seven-ages-of-woman/> (accessed 26 May 2020).

Knight, S. and Edwards, V. (2008) In the company of wolves. *Journal of Aging and Health*, 20: 437–455.

Leist, A. K. (2013) Social media use of older adults: A mini-review. *Gerontology*, 59: 378–384.

Marmot, M. (2015) *The Health Gap*. London: Bloomsbury.

MHA (2020) *Facts and Stats*. Online. HTTP: <www.mha.org.uk/news/policy-influencing/facts-stats/> (accessed 31 August 2020).

Mitas, O., Qian, X., Yarnal, C. and Kerstetter, D. (2011) 'The fun begins now!': Broadening and building processes in Red Hat Society® participation. *Journal of Leisure Research*, 43: 30–55.

Morris, M. C. (2018) *Diet for the Mind: The Latest Science on What to Eat to Prevent Alzheimer's' and Cognitive Decline*. New York: Macmillan.

Mortimer, J. (2016) *No One Should Have No One*. London: Age UK.

The Musical Breath (2020) *Home*. Online. HTTP: <www.themusicalbreath.com/> (accessed 14 August 2020).

National Institute on Aging (2019) *Social Isolation, Loneliness in Older People Pose Health Risks*. Online. HTTP: <www.nia.nih.gov/news/social-isolation-loneliness-older-people-pose-health-risks> (accessed 11 May 2020).

National Institute of Health and Care Excellence (2012) Clinical Guidelines No. 138: 6: Knowing the patient as an individual. In: *Patient Experience in Adult NHS Services: Improving the Experience of Care for People Using Adult NHS Services*. London: Royal College of Physicians.

Nelson-Kakulla, B. (2020) *Gaming Trends of the 50+*. Washington, DC: AARP Research.

New Economics Foundation (2020) *Five Ways to Wellbeing at a Time of Social Distancing*. Online. HTTP: <https://neweconomics.org/2020/03/five-ways-to-wellbeing-at-a-time-of-social-distancing> (accessed 26 May 2020).

Nichols, H. (2017) *What Happens to the Brain as We Age?* Online. HTTP: <www.medical newstoday.com/articles/319185> (accessed 26 May 2020).

Nimrod, G. (2010) The fun culture in seniors' online communities. *The Gerontologist*, 51 (2): 226–237.

Office for National Statistics (2017) *Families and Households in the UK: 2017*. Online. HTTP: <www.ons.gov.uk/peoplepopulationandcommunity/birthsdeathsandmarriages/families/ bulletins/familiesandhouseholds/2017> (accessed 22 November 2020).

Open Access Scotland (2017) *Table Tennis Scotland Batting for Dementia*. Online. HTTP: <www.openaccessgovernment.org/table-tennis-scotland-batting-dementia/40617/> (accessed 20 September 2020).

Outley, C. W. and McKenzie, S. (2006) Older African American women: An examination of the intersections of an adult play group and life satisfaction. *Activities, Adaptation and Aging*, 31: 19–36.

Philip, K., Lewis, A. and Hopkinson, N. S. (2019) Music and dance in chronic lung disease. *Breathe*, 15: 116–120.

Public Health England (2019) *Health Matters: Prevention: A Life Course Approach*. Online. HTTP: <www.gov.uk/government/publications/health-matters-life-course-approach-to-prevention/health-matters-prevention-a-life-course-approach> (accessed 21 November 2020).

Regan, L. and Chi, Y.-L. (2020) *The Indirect Health Effects of COVID-19: Lockdown Measures and Service Provision*. Online. HTTP: <www.cgdev.org/blog/indirect-health-effects-covid-19-lockdown-measures-and-service-provision> (accessed 22 September 2020).

Richardson, J. (2018) *I Am Connected: New Approaches to Supporting People in Later Life Online*. Centre for Ageing Better and Good Things Foundation. Online. HTTP: <www. ageing-better.org.uk/sites/default/files/2018-06/i-am-connected-good-things.pdf> (accessed 20 May 2020).

Rigby, J. (2013) *Why Ping Pong Just Might Be the Elixir of Youth*. Online. HTTP: <www. channel4.com/news/ping-pong-table-tennis-film-dementia-older-people-elixir> (accessed 20 September 2020).

Royal Academy of Dance (2020) *Silver Swans*. Online. HTTP: <www.royalacademyofdance. org/silverswans/> (accessed 14 May 2020).

Scottish Ballet (2020) *Dance, Health and Wellbeing*. Online. HTTP: <www.scottishballet. co.uk/join-in/dance-health-wellbeing> (accessed 28 May 2020).

Stenner, B. J., Buckley, J. D. and Mosewich, A. D. (2020) Reasons why older adults play sport: A systematic review. *Journal of Sport and Health Sciences*, 9 (6): 530–541.

Sutton-Smith, B. (1997) *The Ambiguity of Play*. Cambridge, MA: Harvard University Press.

Tonkin, A. and Whitaker, J. (2020) *Play and Playfulness for Health and Wellbeing: A Panacea for Mitigating the Impact of Coronavirus (COVID 19)*. Online. HTTP: <http://dx.doi. org/10.2139/ssrn.3584412> (accessed 15 September 2020).

U.S. Department of Health and Human Services, Administration for Community Living (2018) *2017 Profile of Older Americans*. Online. HTTP: <https://acl.gov/sites/default/ files/Aging%20and%20Disability%20in%20America/2017OlderAmericansProfile.pdf> (accessed 11 May 2020).

Valtorta, N. K., Kanaan, M., Gilbody, S., Ronzi, S. and Hanratty, B. (2016) Loneliness and social isolation as risk factors for coronary heart disease and stroke: Systematic review and meta-analysis of longitudinal observational studies. *Heart*, 102: 1009–1016.

Vseteckova, J. (2019) *Five Pillars of Aging Well*. Online. HTTP: <www.open.edu/open-learn/health-sports-psychology/mental-health/five-pillars-ageing-well> (accessed 26 May 2020).

West, G. L., Zendel, B. R., Konishi, K., Benady-Chorney, J., Bohbot, V. D., Peretz, I. and Belleville, S. (2017) Playing Super Mario 64 increases hippocampal grey matter in older adults. *PLoS ONE*, 12 (12): e0187779.

Whiteside, B. (2017) *Dance for Parkinson's Scotland (DfPS): A Partnership between Dance Base and Scottish Ballet: Evaluation Report*. Glasgow: Royal Conservatoire of Scotland.

Windle, C., Francis, J. and Coomber, C. (2011) *SCIE Research Briefing 39: Preventing Loneliness and Social Isolation: Interventions and Outcomes*. Online. HTTP: <www.scie.org.uk/prevention/connecting/loneliness-social-isolation-research-2011> (accessed 12 May 2020).

Wood, L., Martin, K., Christian, H., Nathan, A., Lauristen, C., Houghton, S., Kawachi, I. and McCune, S. (2015) The pet factor: Companion animals as a conduit for getting to know people, friendship formation and social support. *PLoS ONE*, 10 (4): e0122085.

World Health Organization (2020) *World Health Statistics 2020: Monitoring Health for the SDGs*. Online. HTTP: <https://apps.who.int/iris/bitstream/handle/10665/332070/9789240005105-eng.pdf?ua=> (accessed 16 May 2020).

Wright, C. (2019) *Think Retirement Is Smooth Sailing? A Look at Its Potential Effects on the Brain*. Online. HTTP: <https://ideas.ted.com/think-retirement-is-smooth-sailing-a-look-at-its-potential-effects-on-the-brain/> (accessed 26 May 2020).

Wright, S. and Wadsworth, A. (2014) Gray and green revisited: A multidisciplinary perspective of gardens, gardening, and the aging process. *Journal of Aging Research*, 2014 (1): 283682.

Yarnal, C. (2006) The Red Hat Society®: Exploring the role of play, liminality, and communitas in older women's lives. *Journal of Women and Aging*, 18: 51–73.

Zhang, F. and Kaufman, D. (2016) Cognitive benefits of older adults' digital gameplay: A critical review. *Gerontechnology*, 15 (1): 3–16.

9 The end of life

In Shakespearean times, people's lives were short: the average life expectancy was around 30 years, and about half of all children died by the age of 15 due to an uncertain food supply, poor hygiene, and limited medical knowledge (Flores 1997). Those who survived childhood might live to 50 or 60 years (Lambert 2020), but it was a relatively small number who reached Shakespeare's stage of 'second childishness' (Shakespeare 2006).

In the 400 years since Shakespeare's death in 1616, at the age of 52, the prospects of appearing in 'the last scene of all' have greatly improved. The number of very elderly people living in the West has increased exponentially, a trend matched in eastern hemisphere nations such as Japan (Mari 2019) and Korea, which has seen the highest increase in their elderly population in the world (Lee et al. 2018). At the start of the twentieth century, the average lifespan in the UK was still only 46 years: today it has reached 81 (Office for National Statistics n.d.). Even more remarkable is the doubling, each year since 1960, of the number of people in Europe and the West living to celebrate their hundredth birthday (Mari 2019).

Daniela Mari (2019) and her team at the University of Milan have been researching the factors at play in this super-aging phenomenon and have uncovered something astounding. As well as evidence for the unsurprising importance of diet, sleep, and exercise, it has emerged that individuals who reach the age of 100 demonstrate a high level of personal resilience which seems 'to make them impervious to the passing of time' (*ibid.*: 114). A study of 119 individuals aged between 97 and 105 concluded that this high level of resilience is linked to the ability to adapt to age-related challenges (Jopp et al. 2016). These findings match those from research into 'Super-Aging' conducted by Northwestern University (2020) which highlights optimism, resilience, and perseverance – as well as active and engaged lifestyles – as key to reaching the end stage of life with aplomb. It is plausible that a lifetime habit of play acts as a viability variable which 'genetically refreshes or fructifies our other, more general, being' and that 'a general feeling of viability is [an] evolutionary salute to play' (Sutton-Smith 2008: 97).

Playing the end game

The super-aging phenomenon has necessitated the recategorization of older adulthood because of a wide variation in the clinical characteristics of the elderly at different ages (Lee et al. 2018). Those aged between 65 and 74 years are defined as the 'youngest-old', those between 75 and 84 years are referred to as 'middle-old', and those above 85 years of age are the 'oldest-old' (Lee et al. 2018). This is important because, as aging progresses, pathophysiologic changes occur more often and 'chronic illnesses, muscular weakness and deterioration of cognitive function' become ever more present (Lee et al. 2018: 249). It also means that the experience of dying in older age will vary, and death will be experienced differently, dependent upon how levels of frailty manifest themselves (Fleming 2016).

Frailty is a clinical condition that develops as a consequence of these pathophysiologic changes (Clegg et al. 2013), when 'multiple body systems gradually lose their in-built reserves', leaving those in a frail state at increasing risk of poor health outcomes, even after a relatively minor event such as a change of medication or environment, or an infection (British Geriatrics Society 2020). Although the precise mechanism associated with frailty is uncertain, there is evidence that physiological reserve can be built up over a lifetime to compensate for later age-related changes (Clegg et al. 2013), as discussed in Chapter 8. While increasing frailty of body and mind cannot ultimately be avoided, this does not imply a necessary frailty of spirit. Durbanville (1957: 25), writing in praise of old age, advises:

> The most important thing is to cultivate a cheerful spirit, never allowing pessimism to gain the upper hand. Make up your mind to maintain a buoyant outlook on life. When the sun shines, let it shine on you. . . . Hang onto your sense of humour with both hands. The older you grow, the more you will need it.

In the following case-story about her 'Uncle Ronnie', Liz Wilkinson describes how a positive outlook and sense of humor can override physical infirmity and allow for the emergence of hidden talents.

Box 9.1 Ronnie Gregan, editor of *Lampoon Weekly*

Elizabeth Wilkinson

Ronnie was a successful businessman, an ironmonger who was highly regarded within that trade throughout Scotland. He has always been deeply respected for his intelligence, humor, and social engagement by his family, friends, local community, and all those with whom he came into contact. Ronnie has achieved this position of social esteem despite a harsh upbringing in a deprived area of Glasgow and the premature death of his wife which left him a lone parent to five children.

Although well cared for physically, Ronnie rarely received any demonstration of affection or praise from his own parents. He was bright and innovative from an early age but nothing he did was ever valued. He received little guidance as far as his education was concerned and, due to the class system at the time, was denied the opportunity to study at a good school. On completing his national service, he was simply expected to join the family business, regardless of any personal aspirations of his own.

After retirement, Ronnie enjoyed a lively social life with a wide circle of friends. His many interests include golf, music, local history, church, and family, and his active involvement in these pursuits meant that he was rarely at home. Several heart attacks failed to dampen Ronnie's spirits and he managed to maintain an active social life through the years. However, a bout of illness two years ago has left him unable to walk without the aid of a Zimmer Frame and means that he is effectively housebound for the first time in his life. But, at the age of 86, Ronnie's spirit remains buoyant. Rather than succumb to despondency, he has honed his creative skills to publish a newspaper, the 'Lampoon Weekly', which is distributed amongst his friends, many of whom are in a similar situation due to their age.

Ronnie structures his day to start work on the paper after breakfast and continues until 4 p.m. He edits articles from current newspapers, adding his own brand of zany humor by cutting and pasting (with scissors and glue!) various cartoons and his own original drawings. The weekly topics are adapted to relate to circumstances and situations pertinent to his readers. This creativity, which was evident but stifled in childhood, has been ever present in his social activities and now, due to enforced immobility, at last has a chance to blossom.

The circulation list for the 'Lampoon Weekly' is gradually dwindling, but Ronnie has vowed to keep going as long as there is someone alive to appreciate his efforts. The process of editing the paper keeps his own spirits aloft and, even when reflecting on his harsh childhood and the missed opportunities, he can quickly turn this around by focusing on the funny side of life. Humor helps to deflect his thoughts from painful memories; rather than wallow in self-pity, he has been able to reflect on his youth, reconciling his inner child issues to release natural talents that have been stifled for so many decades.

Ronnie tells a good story and loves nothing more than a good joke – although he's always quick to say, 'that was nothing like a good joke!' Even when his audience have heard the same stories and jokes many times before, his delivery and infectious laughter has everyone in stitches. His humor draws people to him, averting loneliness and isolation, as Ronnie continues to spread joy to anyone lucky enough to come into his orbit.

Nowadays, the bleakness of 'sans everything' by which Shakespeare defined the 'last scene of all' can be mitigated for. While 'magic bullets don't exist' (Arts for Health 2011), engagement with the creative self at any stage of life allows us to transcend the brutal reality of the ultimate parting and to face the passage between life and death. Hamilton (cited in All-Party Parliamentary Group on Arts, Health and Wellbeing 2017: 142) notes that 'The desire to be creative and feel life is meaningful can be vibrant until the end of life, in spite of physical constraints and mental challenges'. The ability to play is an attribute which defies age limitations and can transform the experience of frailty in the closing years. The following two, quite different, case-stories describe how opportunities for playful connection at the end of life can introduce moments of pure pleasure, nurturing fortitude, and acceptance both in the individual and in those who care for them.

Box 9.2 Pops

Anonymous

Affectionately known as Pops, after being so named by his young granddaughter, our father was the archetypal child of the Second World War. Brought up in an era of rationing and National Service, he spent two years as a Physical Fitness Instructor in the RAF before spending over 30 years as a police officer. Fit and active throughout his life, he was a regular smoker from the age of seven years of age, when he was caught by his mother smoking a cigarette up the chimney.

Pops slowed down post retirement, spending much time in the garden growing vegetables and sweet peas which he would give away, but at the age of 82 he began to have trouble with his legs. The next five years would see constant trips to the hospital as walking became painful and breathing ever more labored. The final two years of Pop's life were spent in and out of hospital – eight weeks in followed by six weeks out before going back in again due to poor circulation which caused the breakdown of the skin and necessitated regular bandaging and re-bandaging of his legs.

Maben et al. (cited in Weldon and Weldon 2016) discuss the coping mechanisms of nursing staff looking after elderly patients. Patients needing complex care, or deemed 'difficult', were described as 'parcels', whereas patients who garnered sympathy and connected with staff were described as 'poppets'. Pops was definitely a poppet.

Pops had always enjoyed singing, and when in hospital, he would serenade the nurses and tell them jokes whenever they were with him. This was a particularly effective ploy when he needed to have his dressings changed. Pops never complained and would often apologize when the nurses found it hard to remove the dressings. He had a simple system for dealing with the pain – the more it hurt, the louder he would sing, trying to get the nurses to sing along as they worked together to get the dressings changed.

At home, he was equally loved by 'his' nurses from the District Nursing Team and the team of lovely carers who looked after our parents.

Knowing how busy they were, there was always a cold can of drink in the fridge for anyone who wanted to take it away with them, along with mounds of chocolate hidden around the bedroom. Visits to the home by the family GP were a special occasion, and the longstanding relationship built up over many years with both our parents was founded on humor and fun (Figure 9.1).

Toward the end, inhibitions gradually disappeared as dementia set in, but this just revealed a more wicked sense of humor, especially after a dose of morphine had been administered. Pops' singing was robust, and the performance of jokes louder than usual, until the sleepiness kicked in and an hour or so of pain-free slumber ensued, allowing peace to return to the house.

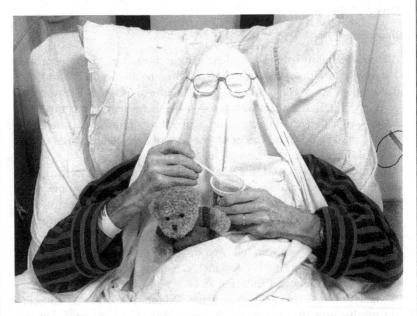

Figure 9.1 Pops during a typical hospital visit

Source: Photograph by Alison Tonkin.

Box 9.3 Playful objects in advanced dementia care

Cathy Treadaway

One of the greatest difficulties in caring for people in the advanced stages of dementia is their withdrawal from the world. The disease severely impacts memory, perception, and verbal communication; in the later stages, speech may be lost altogether. At this stage it is also difficult for a person to initiate activity. Finding playful ways of stimulating them and keeping their interest in the world around them is vital to their care. Providing social connection, comfort, and sensory stimulation through playful objects can have a huge positive benefit for a person's wellbeing. Our LAUGH (n.d.) research project, funded by the UK Arts and Humanities Research Council, was aimed to develop a range of playful handheld objects to increase the wellbeing of people living with advanced dementia. Currently, very few products exist that are designed for people at this stage of the disease. The aim was to design playful objects informed by the expertise of health and care professionals and developed in collaboration with people living with advanced dementia. This is the story of one of the playful objects we designed for a lady who was in the final stages of the disease and who was considered by her carers to be on 'end of life care'.

Thelma was 93 years old when the LAUGH design team met her. She was no longer able to speak, was bed-bound, and when she did get out of bed, she frequently fell. Her hands were stiff and contorted, and she had lost her appetite and desire to socialize. When we asked about the kind of thing we could design for her, the carers said that all she really needed at this stage in her life was a hug. The team decided to use this as a starting point for developing a new product that would give Thelma comfort in her final days.

The team designed HUG™, a soft wearable object to be cuddled, reminiscent of a soft doll, cushion, and teddy. HUG™ contains a simulated beating heart and a microcontroller with speakers that can be programmed to play a person's favorite music playlist or a story, or poetry etc. The object has long 'arms' and 'legs' that are weighted at the ends and, when wrapped around a person, gives them the sensation of being hugged. The aim was to create the experience of both giving and receiving a hug.

The day HUG™ was first given to Thelma, she barely opened her eyes but nestled down into it and listened to the music, clearly finding pleasure in the softness of the body. When the researchers returned a week later, Thelma was much more alert, and carers reported that she was enjoying HUG™ and had seemed a little better. Over the course of the following three months there was a continued and significant improvement in Thelma's health and wellbeing. She began to eat again, was out of bed, her speech returned, and she was more willing to socialize, her hands relaxed, and she regained movement in her fingers. Most significant of all, Thelma did not fall again after she had been given HUG™. The playful object was her baby, something to care for and love, and a reason to continue to live. Thelma lived happily for a further nine months with improved general health and quality of life. HUG™ has subsequently been evaluated in a much larger trial

which has corroborated its benefits to wellbeing for people living with
advanced dementia (Hume 2019).

Finding playful ways to engage people in the advanced stages of
dementia is vital for maintaining their quality of life. Playfulness happens
in the moment, and activities and objects that promote playful experiences
can provide comfort, connection, and pleasure when a person's memory
and cognition are compromised by the disease.

Aging is accompanied by structural and physiological alterations in the brain
which are responsible for functional change, and frailty is associated with a
faster rate of cognitive decline (Clegg et al. 2013). Reducing frailty is of benefit
to society as a whole, but even more importantly to the individual and their
family. There is growing interest in strategies to delay or mitigate the impact
of the aging process (British Geriatrics Society 2020), particularly in relation
to the brain. Cognitive reserve refers to 'the idea that people develop a reserve
of thinking abilities during their lives, and that this protects them against losses
that can occur through ageing and disease', building resilience that can be
called upon in later life (Stern 2020). Educational and occupational attainment
as well as engagement with leisure activities throughout the life course seem to
have a protective effect on cognitive reserve (*ibid.* 2012), suggesting that 'cognitive engagement provides cognitive reserve that delays the onset of cognitive
impairment' (Anderson 2015). As suggested by Stern (2020), it is 'never too
late to start, and the more activities the better: the effect appears to be cumula-
tive'. Playful endeavors, especially those which incorporate elements of novelty
and challenge, are limitless and, when freely motivated, add value at any age
(Perry et al. 2000).

Playful preparation for life's ending

Play at the end of life, as in the preceding years, is principally a source of
healthful pleasure: arousing and becalming in equal measure. It maintains and
develops our connections to others and to our inner selves. Outside of time,
play occupies a space all of its own, elevating the player above the actuality of
their lived experience. At the end of life, play allows us to enter the ultimate
'zone of authenticity' (Whitaker and Tonkin 2019), where the trappings of
everyday life are stripped away, and we are free to become purely and completely ourselves.

John Killick (2012: 15) describes play as 'the unfettering of mind and body',
manifest in childhood as 'a natural response to the awareness of being alive in
the senses'. In adulthood, opportunities for such 'unfettering' are more elusive
but, when personal and societal constraints and expectations can be cast aside,
the rediscovery of play can enrich our experience of living in the world in

all its aspects. As we move through our later years toward life's conclusion, it is possible once again to embrace the joy of simply being alive, released from societal demands and conventions to become our authentic selves (Mengers 2014).

Children play with the concept of death all the time: the notions of 'being' and 'unbeing' are evident in their early play (Whitaker and Tonkin 2019) and reemerge throughout childhood. In adolescence, the belief in personal immortality characteristic of youth is evident in the death-defying and death-denying games popular among the young (Wenk 2010).

For many children and young people, their first real experience of human loss and bereavement comes with the death of a grandparent or an elderly relative. Throughout recent history, stories have been used to introduce children to the subject of death (Butler 1972) using metaphor and analogy. In recent decades, children's literature has taken a more realistic turn (Moore and Mae 2006), and there has been a proliferation of books aimed at helping children to understand and cope with loss. One example is *Cry, Heart, But Never Break* (Ringtved 2016), in which death is portrayed as a storyteller who prepares the children for the impending loss of their grandmother. The simplicity of the message that grief and sorrow are necessary before life can move on provides a platform for further exploration of death and dying in a gentle and age- appropriate manner. Death is a prominent feature of Young Adult fiction and author Rupert Wallis (2014) argues that this is important because it helps young people 'to consider how death shapes life; not only in the philosophical sense of grappling with the nature of existence but also practically, in terms of how to live, how to be'.

In contrast to the efforts of the literary world to confront the reality of death head on, the digital games industry encourages and extends an immature concept of death as impermanent and avoidable. Yee et al. (2019) explored the impact of exposure to violent video games on Malaysian Chinese children aged between 10 and 12 years and found that increased exposure to these games was matched by a corresponding decrease in fear of death and an increase in the belief that death is reversible and can be avoided. Even nonviolent games have been shown to skew perceptions of death. The hugely popular world of SIMS™, is a life simulation game played by both children and adults, which involves the creation of virtual characters whose lives and lifestyles are determined by the player (EA Games 2020). In the SIMS 4 Death Guide which identifies ways of cheating death, characters can be resurrected, countering death from 'basic and preventable fires, to the (kind of) inevitable old age, and unchecked emotional extremes' (Carl's Guides 2020). Sims can also die from emotional extremes, one of which is being too playful, whereby the character laughs themselves to death, unless it calms down or goes to sleep (*ibid.*). These games reinforce the idea that death is impermanent and can be manipulated, resulting in a distorted perception of the world and reinforcing death as a societal taboo (Yee et al. 2019).

It is typically our first real-life encounter with death that leads to the full realization that we cannot control or sustain our own lives. Baars (2016) says that 'death is part of our lives as soon as we *know* that we will die: This knowledge has consequences, even if we repress or deny it'. The revelation of our own mortality is a fact so profound that it is suppressed, and we develop defense mechanisms to avoid confronting the ultimate truth (Florian and Mikulincer 2004). This was seen during the 2020 coronavirus pandemic as people struggled to process their emotional reactions to the crisis (Kessler cited in Burns 2020). However, Firestone (2018) concedes that some defenses can have positive benefits, such as 'the symbolic immortality that is fostered by the imagination of living on through creative works in art, literature, and science' as well as 'finding lasting meaning in devotion to family, friends, and people at large, and attempting to leave a positive legacy'.

We eventually have to face the reality of our own death and to experience and communicate the accompanying emotions in some way. In his final broadcast interview, the playwright Dennis Potter (cited in Rockwell 1994) shared the following insight:

> We're the one animal that knows that we're going to die, and yet we carry on paying our mortgages, doing our jobs, moving about, behaving as though there's eternity in a sense, and we tend to forget that life can only be defined in the present tense. It is, and it is now only.

Baars (2016) speaks of the need to 'practice dying' as a way of learning how to live a finite life; finding the courage to anticipate loss can reveal the richness of possibilities in our present 'finite' lives.

In *The Top Five Regrets of the Dying – A Life Transformed by the Dearly Departing*, Bronnie Ware (2019) draws on her many years' experience working in palliative care to share how she has transformed her own life as a result of the lessons she has learned from the dying. Ware itemizes the five most common end-of-life regrets: (1) I wish I'd had the courage to live a life true to myself, not the life others expected of me; (2) I wish I hadn't worked so hard; (3) I wish I'd had the courage to express my feelings; (4) I wish I had stayed in touch with my friends; and (5) I wish that I had let myself be happier. She argues that it is resistance to the idea of our own mortality that denies us the opportunity to live truly authentic lives.

Play has been a feature of cultural practices related to dying and death since ancient times: art, music, dance, theater, play, contemplation, rituals, and somatic practices (Fox and McDermott 2020). A growing recognition of the need to find new ways to explore the concept of death 'as a natural part of life – both necessary and inevitable' (Ringtved 2016) is reflected in a unique enterprise by the Academy of Medical Sciences (2019). In the following case-story, Nick Hillier describes this innovative project, illustrating how a playful approach can be used to open the door on a difficult topic.

Box 9.4 Welcome to the Departure Lounge. How opening a shop helped people to understand death

Nick Hillier

Death is a destination for all of us, a journey we will all make, and just like our holiday travel experiences – our experience of death will be different depending on how prepared or unprepared we are.

To explore the public's views on the of role medical research in preparing people for the end of life, the Academy of Medical Sciences working in collaboration with design agency, The Liminal Space, opened 'The Departure Lounge' in an empty shop in Lewisham Shopping Centre, London in May/June 2019 (Figure 9.2).

Using the metaphor of travel, we played with cultural references and expectations in an attempt to translate and communicate information about the end of life in a way that made people feel safe and comfortable. This created a space where unusually open conversations about life, death, loss, and family occurred.

The journey to the Departure Lounge started with large window posters that looked like holiday ads – but actually introduced the topic of dying. This strange juxtaposition attracted attention and got people talking and asking questions, even if they didn't enter the 'shop'.

We continued to play with the power of the unexpected, through the display of a huge pile of luggage (Figure 9.3), each suitcase bearing luggage tags with key statistics and information points, as well as stories of lived experiences. Video screens picked up on visual references from these stories and a soundscape filled the space. This was not just to bring the stories to life, but to ensure that the Departure Lounge wasn't a silent and somber place.

Visitors commented that they came in to browse the suitcases, then had a gradual realization that they portrayed stories about the end of life. This unexpected and lighthearted shift, and the curious feeling of matter out of place, somehow offset their reluctance to talk about dying.

At the back of the shop, we created a life-sized departures board. Each square on the board formed a box that could be opened to find answers to frequently asked questions about end-of-life matters. The answers were printed on objects, including travel slippers, passport holders, eye masks, and boarding cards that visitors could touch, hold, and play with while they interacted with the space.

A light installation, designed to resemble the airport windows which travelers walk past on route to the departure gate, provided a space for visitors to record their hopes for their final journey or the memory of a loved one's death.

Three 'departure gates' marked the point where visitors could sit down for in-depth conversations with shop guides from a range of backgrounds – not just researchers and healthcare professionals, but also people with experience of caring for loved ones at the end of life. We included another private space in the shop where people could spend time, should any of the content trigger difficult memories or feelings.

Following their visit, people recognized that it is important to overcome the taboo and talk about death; that emotions and cultural norms make it difficult; and that it is important to prepare for the end of life by letting loved ones know your wishes.

For some people, their visit to the Departure Lounge bore witness to their experiences of death and dying, and even provided solace for those living with end-of-life care dilemmas and grief. Visitors had experiences that were emotionally impactful, and the content led to a recognition that thinking about death and end-of-life care is important because there are choices that can be made.

Unsurprisingly the need to explore 'what matters to you?' and not 'what's the matter with you?' was a really common theme of discussions. We heard time and time again that a good death was one that allowed someone to be surrounded by the people they loved, doing the things they loved most, for as long as possible. Very often, this was about being able to have a glass of their favorite tipple! But the underlying message was that the best care will let that happen, even if it means bending the rules just a little bit.

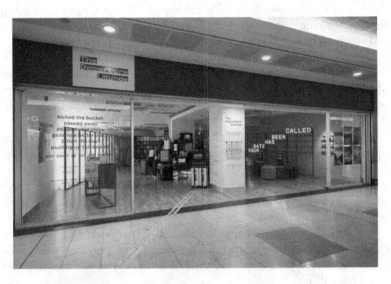

Figure 9.2 The Departure Lounge shop front

Source: Photograph by Ashley Bingham for The Liminal Space.

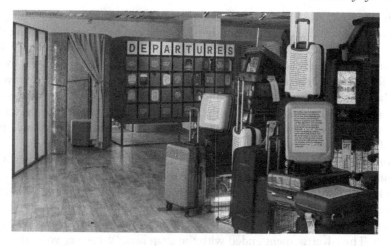

Figure 9.3 Suitcases as playful and informative artifacts

Source: Photograph by Ashley Bingham for The Liminal Space.

How we die involves a profoundly personal journey and each individual approaches the matter of death in a highly personal way. The success of the Departure Lounge rests in its broad reach, combining factual information, personal narrative, and symbolic imagery in the safe and familiar context of the local high street. The following example of evaluative feedback from one of the visitors to the Departure Lounge reinforces the point.

> You've got stats, you've got academic, you've got more personal – literally personal handwriting, you've got visual, you've got random arty things with the suitcase labels, you've got the postcards so it's just multidimensional. You take that and you think of a new way to broach it with my family – maybe I'm not broaching that subject in the way that's suitable for them. Maybe there's another way to do it. The exhibit helps with that.

Swiss psychiatrist, Elisabeth Kubler-Ross (2008) is widely attributed with changing attitudes to talking about death by encouraging health professionals to be more honest with themselves and with their patients when they are approaching the end of life. Kubler-Ross may have changed the way the medical profession approaches the subject of death and dying, but the lessons learned have been slow to filter through to society at large. Research by Age UK (n.d.) in 2018 found that 36 per cent of people are still uncomfortable raising the subject of death with family or friends, although a survey by the Cooperative Society in 2019 found that reluctance to talk about death and dying had reduced slightly to 16.5 million in 2019 from 18 million the previous year (Cooperative Group Limited 2019). In the words of O'Mahony (2016: 55), 'death hasn't quite come out of the closet, but its toe is sticking out'.

In the UK, the charity *Dying Matters* (2020a) continues to advocate for people to talk more openly about dying, death, and bereavement, stating that a lack of openness and our reluctance to talk about death has 'affected our ability to die where or how we would wish'. In a blog for the digital media platform *Death Matters*, Luscomb (2018) writes: 'Dead is a four letter word. Perhaps that is why it is not uttered in polite company'. When the right words are hard to find, the creative use of play and playfulness can help to overcome the strong personal and social resistance to making death an acceptable part of life.

In 2018, the Marie Curie Charity launched a public health television advertisement which used humor to describe common euphemisms associated with death. The advert featured a song accompanied by visual graphics to illustrate terms such as 'fall off the perch', 'kick the bucket', 'shuffle off this mortal coil' (another phrase penned by Shakespeare), and 'meet your maker' (Wheaton 2019). The advertisement ended with the strap line, 'Whatever you call it, we should talk about it', inviting people to engage in conversations that explore their own death or the death of a loved one (Wheaton 2019).

Dying Matters promotes the use of end-of-life games to prompt conversations, featuring a board game called Circle of Life and a simple card game called The Conversation Game (Dying Matters 2020b). It is becoming increasingly acceptable to adopt such a playful approach to engaging in conversation about death with a 'virtual avalanche of card and board games that prompt participants to talk about death' (Clohessy 2020). Games such as the board games *Bucket List, Death Insight and Conversation Cards, Elephant in the Room, Morbid Curiosity*, and *The Death Deck* all aim to facilitate conversations in which people can talk about what matters most to them in the present and what will matter to them most when their life comes to an end.

The Death Café (n.d.) movement is another seriously playful approach to reframing the subject of death, fostering open conversation in a convivial atmosphere, helped along by tea and cake. Festivals such as the Joy of Death Festival (Williams 2012), the Festival of Death and Dying (2019), and York's Dead Good Festival (n.d.) incorporate art, theatre, film, and music-making in lively attempts to celebrate death as part of life. US Broadcaster and palliative care consultant, Terry Gross (cited in Clohessy 2020) opines: 'The increasing variety of new entry points (games, festivals, feasts, cafes, etc.) that invite people into conversations about what matters most at the end of life is unquestionably helping our society engage in a conversation that had become taboo'.

Play at life's ending

Killick (2012: 16) cites Nachmanovitch's definition of the Sanskrit word for play which also translates as 'delight and enjoyment of this moment' and, at the end of life's days, the concept of 'this moment' acquires a unique poignancy. A study by Dönmez and Johnston (2020) explores what it means to those approaching the end of their lives to 'live in the moment', isolating five attributes most commonly associated with this concept, namely: *enjoying simple pleasures, prioritizing relationships, living each day to the fullest, maintaining normality,* and *not worrying about the future.* There is evident correlation between these characteristics and some of the features of play, most notably the pleasure derived from intrinsically motivated experiences and their positive consequences in terms of positive reframing and enhanced coping. Play 'in the moment' comes to represent a creative bridge between the two levels of human experience: the tangible and the intangible, the surface and the deep (Kearney 1997). In the words of Brian Sutton-Smith: 'play [is] at heart always a kind of transcendence' (2008: 96).

All forms of creative expression are inherently transformative; a tangible conveyance of personal insights, ideas, or feelings (Newton 1961). As an example of 'deep play', the creative arts communicate essential truths beneath a veil of 'submerged metaphors, images, actions, personalities, jokes' (Ackerman 1999: 122). The All-Party Parliamentary Group (APPG) on Arts, Health and Wellbeing (2017) reference the contribution made by the Arts at the end of life. The artist, Perry Grayson describes how

> art helps us access and express parts of ourselves that are often unavailable to other forms of human interaction. It flies below the radar, delivering nourishment for our soul and returning with stories from the unconscious. . . . Art, like science and religion, helps us make meaning from our lives, and to make meaning is to make us feel better.
>
> (Grayson, cited in APPG on Arts,
> Health and Wellbeing 2017: Introduction)

The British visual artist, Edward Dutkiewicz (1961–2007) is best known for his use of bright colors and abstract forms. Following his death from multiple sclerosis, the collector Michael Estorick, wrote:

> [I]f there are echoes of Alexander Calder and Matisse in his use of bright colour and abstract form, it is also of their playfulness and joy. For sure, no one who has experienced so much pain has also expressed as much fun and the pleasure of simply being alive, or, for that matter, has given so much to those around him.
>
> (Karia 2020)

As a means of creative self-expression – whether through art, music, reminiscence, or simply being present in the moment – play can facilitate a return to the awareness of 'being alive in the senses' (Killick 2012) and reveal the possibility of meeting death with joy (Twycross 1997).

The 'Art of Behalf' approach described by Ganzon et al. (2020), for example, reveals how a co-created 'artistic reflection of a patient's story in a time of uncertainty and loss can help affirm the patient's value as a person and what is meaningful to their life' and so contribute to a sense of 'unified narrative identity' at life's ending (De Lange 2014: 516). A similar premise underlies *Lifesongs* (Academy for the Love of Learning 2020), an intergenerational arts program which uses various art forms, including storytelling, music, and poetry to validate the experiences of people in elderly care and hospices, embedding them at the heart of a creative community. The idea of 'communion' – as an act or instance of intimate togetherness – is also fundamental to The Threshold Choir (2020), a global movement of singers who use their collective voices to connect with individuals 'on the threshold' of living and dying. Simple songs and lullabies with short, repetitive refrains are used 'to communicate ease, comfort and presence', elevating a moment of transition from its mundane reality to a place of oneness and wholeness.

The Dutch charity, *Stichting Ambulance Wens* (Ambulance Wish Foundation), started 13 years ago by ambulance driver Kee Veldoer and his wife Ineke, helps to fulfill wishes for people who are stretcher-bound and terminally ill, many of whom are close to death (Venema 2015). The charity offers the dying one last chance to enjoy simple pleasures, many of which are activities that have previously brought joy to their lives. The wishes have included attendance at weddings and funerals, a longing to see the sea, and a visit to the zoo and an art gallery. Knot, a district nurse who volunteers for the charity (cited in Venema 2015) comments that, whilst it can be emotionally draining to grant final wishes, 'often people are ready to die because they are so far down the line, and then it's nice to give them something they really want'. Lok (cited in Venema 2015), another nursing volunteer, sums up her experiences with the charity stating, 'it has taught me that you can find happiness in the little things, that's what you should aim for – rather than longing for what you don't have'.

However, it remains the case that for most people death remains a medical event which takes place in hospital (O'Mahony 2016) with little opportunity for playful preparation or the granting of last wishes. In 2016, almost half (46.9 per cent) of all deaths took place in hospital with just a quarter (23.5 per cent) occurring in people's own homes; 21.8 per cent of deaths were in care homes and just 5.7 per cent in hospices (Public Health England 2018). O'Mahony (2016) expresses the view that our societal avoidance of death is largely due to it being 'hidden' away in hospitals where it is seen as an affront to medicine's healing focus, making a good death increasingly difficult.

Taking a final bow

When people are able to challenge their emotional defenses and open up in conversations about death, they are in a better position to confront death with equanimity and to end their lives in the way they wish. When society ceases to regard death as a problem to be solved and the process of dying is de-medicalized, we might then be able to fashion a new *ars moriendi* (art of dying) which allows us to bring death out of the closet (O'Mahony 2016). A collective consciousness of existential issues of life and death, and an acceptance of personal vulnerability in relation to the universe, allows for a deeper understanding and respect for our own wellbeing needs and those of others: 'In becoming more open and vulnerable, we are able to more fully embrace love and the spirit of life' (Firestone 2018).

Ware (2020) observes, 'People grow a lot when they are faced with their own mortality. I learnt never to underestimate someone's capacity for growth'. Recognizing that our time on earth is finite, encourages us to live life as fully as possible with an appreciation of all it has to offer. Durbanville (1957) enthuses: 'These are the best years of my life – the sweetest and most free from anxious care. The way grows brighter; the birds sing sweeter; the winds blow softer; the sun shines more radiantly than ever before'. This sentiment is summed up in the words of Potter (cited in Rockwell 1994), who proclaimed, 'the nowness of everything is absolutely wondrous'.

In our last case-story, Julia returns to the theme of reading aloud as a means of satisfying a yearning to connect with her aging mother, describing how books and the gift of reading gave shape and meaning to their last Goodbyes. When it comes to relationships, 'There is no real ending. It's just the place where you stop the story' (Herbert cited in Brown 2020).

Box 9.5 Closing the book: reading aloud in the nursing home

Julia Whitaker

My mother loved books. As a schoolgirl, she read her way through a year's confinement with rheumatic fever and then as a young woman went on to qualify as a children's librarian. In the 1960s, Bernadette set up the Lower School library at King Alfred School (KAS) in North London, where she worked for over 30 years, imparting her love of books and of reading to generations of students. At KAS, the library was so much more than a resource center: a 'nurture hub' long before the term was invented; a refuge for those struggling to cope in the classroom; somewhere for a chat when you could find no one to play with. Whatever your interest, whatever your project, whatever your worry, Bernadette had 'just the book' to meet your need. Our family home too, was filled with stories; books read, discussed, gifted, and exchanged.

It is a cruel irony therefore, that when diagnosed with a form of dementia at the age of 70, one of the first signs was Bernadette's struggle to process the written word. Her beloved books had become a source of frustration and bewilderment. By the time she moved into residential care, I was living 300 miles away, in a new relationship with a new baby, but for the remaining eight years of her life, we traveled to visit 'Grandma' every couple of months. Our luggage bursting with books to tide us through the long journey and the tedious nursing home visits, it was now my turn to return the gift of reading to the mother who had given it to me.

As I read my way through a selection of favorite children's books with my toddler daughter, Grandma would fix us with a 'hard stare' to rival

that of Paddington Bear, murmuring 'Yes, yes' in recognition of a familiar tale. With an infant-like need for sensory feedback, she would reach
out to grab the book, bringing it close to her face to sniff or to kiss, as
if inhaling the memory of a long-lost magic. As the years passed and
Bernadette gradually disappeared into the densening fog of dementia,
it was reading stories that both maintained our connection and created
a new bond with the granddaughter to whom she had never been able
to read herself. Our reading would often rouse Grandma from her stu-
por, evoking a laugh or exclamation – a sign of the life to which she
was stubbornly hanging on. When she became agitated or restless, our
storytelling could still the muscle spasms, presaging a drift into peaceful
slumber. As my mother's days drew to a close, I watched desperately for
these precious indications that she was aware of my presence and, when
they eventually evaporated entirely, I kept on reading, unwilling to let go
of that golden thread of connection.

In *The Enchanted Hour*, Cox Gurdon (2019) cites similar examples of
adult children who have found reading aloud to be a way of reaching out
to parents at the end of their lives. In the same way that sharing stories
nurtures attachment at the start of life, reading to our elderly parents
'shows them that they matter to us, that we want to expand time and
attention and energy' (*ibid.*: 180) in order to make something good of the
'painful crudity and hopeless dreariness' of that ultimate parting (Einstein
cited in Cox Gurdon 2019: 179).

Parting words

Baars (2016) states, 'We do not die because we have become old but because
we have been born as finite human beings: death is given with life'. This
echoes the stoic philosophers, such as Seneca (4 BCE–65 CE), who argued
that the best way to live with death is to simply accept it: since it is unavoid-
able, it is futile to dwell on the matter (*ibid.*). This chimes with Heidegger's
(1996) concept of 'being-towards-death', which rests on the acceptance that
life comes to an end in death, and that the freedom to live an authentic life
derives from accepting the necessity of one's own mortality (Critchley 2009).
With increasing age, people acquire a deeper understanding of human life as a
process of continuous change which demands a constant readiness to question,
to wonder, to begin anew (Baars 2016) – and our personal play history informs
this capacity for adaptation and growth.

Gestalt psychologist, Rudolf Arnheim (1986: 285) uses the metaphor of a
never-ending staircase overlying an arc to represent the endless possibilities of
the human lifespan. The arc represents the biological process of aging, which
starts with a period of growth, followed by 'the unfolded powers' of maturity,
before the onset of progressive decline (Figure 9.4). The staircase symbolizes an

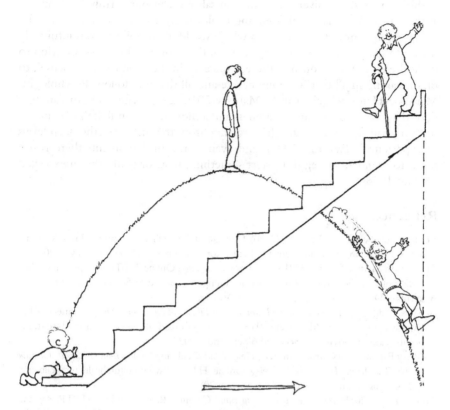

Figure 9.4 Contrasting conceptualizations of the human lifespan

Source: Adapted from Arnheim (1986) by Lizzy Mikietyn.

alternative worldview, of life as an infinite ascent toward wisdom and creativity, which extends beyond 'the confines of our years and our lifetime' (Mari 2019: 115). Play and creativity at life's ending represent the ultimate expression of a lifetime of experiencing what it means to be fully human.

Whether one holds the view that the lifespan has a finite endpoint, or believes that it extends beyond earthly time, it can be argued that there is a place for joy and playfulness at its biological conclusion, as the individual is freed from 'the compulsions of conscience and impulsions of irrationality' (Erikson 1995: 192) to finally experience authentic selfhood.

Conclusion

Reviewing a lifetime spent 'fishing the waters of play theory', Brian Sutton-Smith (2008) reflects: 'Play begins as a major feature of mammalian evolution and remains as a major method of becoming reconciled with our being within our present universe . . . human salvation in our earthly box'. Just as at the start of life, play at life's ending is ultimately a search for meaning. The infant emerges from the womb to a whole world of possibility and is intuitively driven to explore ways of making sense of that world and their connection to it. At the end of life's journey, there is once again the need to 'make sense', to find meaning in all that has gone before and all that will follow. Psychologist, Marie de Hennezel (cited in O'Mahony 2016: 228) writes: 'Death can be a door that opens to a greater awareness and a more meaningful life'. Play in any of its myriad forms facilitates that crossing 'from the surface to the deep levels of experience' (Twycross 1997), and even in the final moments there is still room to wonder, to begin, to start something new, or to do the unexpected (Arendt 1958).

References

Academy for the Love of Learning (2020) *Lifesongs*. Online. HTTP: <https://aloveoflearning. org/academy-programs/institute-for-living-story/lifesongs/> (accessed 5 July 2020).

Academy of Medical Sciences (2019) *The Departure Lounge*. Online. HTTP: <https://acmedsci. ac.uk/policy/policy-projects/the-departure-lounge> (accessed 11 September 2020).

Ackerman, D. (1999) *Deep Play*. New York: Vintage.

Age UK (n.d.) *Why We Should All Be Encouraged to Talk about Death and Dying*. Online. HTTP: <www.ageuk.org.uk/discover/2018/why-we-should-all-be-encouraged-to-talk-about-death-and-dying/> (accessed 6 September 2020).

All Party Parliamentary Group on Arts, Health and Wellbeing (2017) *Inquiry Report: Creative Health: The Arts for Health and Wellbeing*. Online. HTTP: <www.culturehealthandwellbeing. org.uk/appg-inquiry/> (accessed 14 April 2020).

Anderson, N. (2015) *It's Never Too Late to Build Cognitive Reserve*. Online. HTTP: <www. psychologytoday.com/gb/blog/living-mild-cognitive-impairment/201511/building-cognitive-reserve> (accessed 3 September 2020).

Arendt, H. (1958) *The Human Condition*. Chicago: University of Chicago Press.

Arnheim, R. (1986) *New Essays on the Psychology of Art*. Berkley: University of California Press.

Arts for Health (2011) *Arts for Health Manifesto Part One*. Online. HTTP: <www.arts forhealth.org/manifesto/ManifestoPartOne.pdf> (accessed 18 October 2020).

Baars, J. (2016) Aging: Learning to live a finite life. *The Gerontologist*, 57 (5): 969–976.

British Geriatrics Society (2020) *New 'One-Stop Shop' for Frailty*. Online. HTTP: <www. bgs.org.uk/policy-and-media/new-%E2%80%98one-stop-shop%E2%80%99-for-frailty> (accessed 3 September 2020).

Brown, D. (2020, 24 November) Beginnings & endings: A how-to reflection for writers. [Blog]. *The Darling Axe*. Online. HTTP: <https://darlingaxe.com/blogs/news/no-real-ending> (accessed 20 July 2020).

Burns, L. (2020) *Elisabeth Kübler-Ross: The Rise and Fall of the Five Stages of Grief*. Online. HTTP: <www.bbc.co.uk/news/stories-53267505> (accessed 5 September 2020).

Butler, F. (1972) Death in children's literature. *Children's Literature*, 1 (1): 104–124.

Carl's Guides (2020) *The SIMS 4: Death Guide: Preventing Death, Resurrection, and Ways Sims Can Die*. Online. HTTP: <www.carls-sims-4-guide.com/death/> (accessed 13 September 2020).

Clegg, A., Young, J., Iliffe, S., Olde Rikkert, M. and Rockwood, K. (2013) Frailty in older people. *The Lancet*, 2, 381 (9868): 752–762. doi:10.1016/S0140-6736(12)62167-9.

Clohessy, K. (2020) *People Are Playing Games to Help Them Talk about Death*. Online. HTTP: <https://blog.sevenponds.com/something-special/people-are-playing-games-to-help-them-talk-about-death> (accessed 3 September 2020).

Cooperative Group Limited (2019) *Burying Traditions: The Changing Face of UK Funerals*. Online. HTTP: <https://assets.ctfassets.net/iqbixcpmwym2/5v6n2gA1yGR5BCDRJ4kN Ku/93696c8e8e2f9e260795c941fa96c6c9/3876_1_Funeralcare_Media_pack_artwork_ SML_v4.pdf> (accessed 6 September 2020).

Cox Gurdon, M. (2019) *The Enchanted Hour: The Miraculous Power of Reading Aloud in the Age of Distraction*. London: Piakus.

Critchley, S. (2009) *Being and Time Part 6: Death*. Online. HTTP: <www.theguardian.com/ commentisfree/belief/2009/jul/13/heidegger-being-time> (accessed 1 July 2020).

Death Café (n.d.) *Home*. Online. HTTP: <https://deathcafe.com/> (accessed 6 September 2020).

De Lange, D. F. (2014) Affirming life in the face of death: Ricoeur's living up to death as a modern ars moriendi and a lesson for palliative care. *Medicine, Health Care, and Philosophy*, 17 (4): 509–518.

Dönmez, C. F. and Johnston, B. (2020) Living in the moment for people approaching the end of life: A concept analysis. *International Journal of Nursing Studies*, 108: 103584.

Durbanville, H. (1957) *The Best Is Yet to Be*. Edinburgh: McCall Barbour.

Dying Matters (2020a) *About Us*. Online. HTTP: <www.dyingmatters.org/overview/ about-us> (accessed 11 September 2020).

Dying Matters (2020b) *End of Life Games*. Online. HTTP: <www.dyingmatters.org/page/ end-life-games> (accessed 22 November 2020).

EA Games (2020) *SIMS 4*. Online. HTTP: <www.origin.com/gbr/en-us/store/the-sims/ the-sims-4#store-page-section-description> (accessed 13 September 2020).

Erikson, E. H. (1995) *Childhood and Society*. New York: Vintage.

Festival of Death and Dying (2019) *Home*. Online. HTTP: <https://deathfest.co.uk/> (accessed 6 September 2020).

Firestone, R. W. (2018) *Death Anxiety*. Online. HTTP: <www.psychologytoday.com/us/ blog/the-human-experience/201805/death-anxiety> (accessed 4 September 2020).

Fleming, J. (2016) Here's what people in their 90s really think about death. *The Conversation*. Online. HTTP: <https://theconversation.com/heres-what-people-in-their-90s-really-think-about-death-58053> (accessed 3 September 2020).

Flores, S. (1997) *Shakespeare's World*. Online. HTTP: <www.webpages.uidaho.edu/~sflores/ 345world.html> (accessed 6 July 2020).

Florian, V. and Mikulincer, M. (2004) A multifaceted perspective on the existential meanings, manifestations, and consequences of the fear of personal death. In: Greenberg, J., Koole, S. L. and Pyszczynski, T. (Eds.), *Handbook of Experimental Existential Psychology*. New York: Guilford: 54–70.

Fox, K. M. and McDermott, L. (2020) Where is leisure when death is present? *Leisure Sciences*. doi:10.1080/01490400.2020.1774012.

Ganzon, C., O'Callaghan, C. and Dwyer, J. (2020) 'Art on behalf': Introducing an accessible art therapy approach used in palliative care. *The Arts in Psychotherapy*, 67, February: 101616.

Heidegger, M. (1996) *Basic Writings: Martin Heidegger*. Abingdon, Oxon: Routledge.

Hume, C. (2019) *Dementia Device 'Kind of Brought My Mum Back'*. Online. HTTP: <www. bbc.co.uk/news/uk-wales-50237366> (accessed 12 September 2020).

Jopp, D. S., Park, M. S., Lehrfeld, J. and Paggi, M. (2016) Physical, cognitive, social and mental health in near-centenarians and centenarians living in New York City: Findings from the Fordham Centenarian Study. *BMC Geriatrics*, 16 (1).

Karia, A. (2020) *Collection Highlight: Edward Dutkiewicz*. Online. HTTP: <www.painting sinhospitals.org.uk/Blogs/collection/collection-highlight-edward-dutkiewicz> (accessed 5 July 2020).

Kearney, M. (1997) *Mortally Wounded: Stories of Soul, Pain, Death and Healing*. New York: Simon and Schuster.

Killick, J. (2012) *Playfulness and Dementia: A Practice Guide*. London: Jessica Kingsley Publishers.

Kubler-Ross, E. (2008) *On Death and Dying*. Abingdon, Oxon: Routledge.

Lambert, T. (2020) *A Brief History of Life Expectancy in Britain*. Online. HTTP: <www.loc alhistories.org/life.html> (accessed 6 July 2020).

LAUGH (n.d.) *Design for Dementia*. Online. HTTP: <www.laughproject.info/> (accessed 12 September 2020).

Lee, S. B., Oh, J. H., Park, J. H., Choi, S. P. and Wee, J. H. (2018) Differences in youngest-old, middle-old, and oldest-old patients who visit the emergency department. *Clinical and Experimental Emergency Medicine*, 5 (4): 249–255. doi.org/10.15441/ceem.17.261.

Luscomb, D. (2018) *Discussion*. Online. HTTP: <https://deathmatters.ca/the-d-word/> (accessed 4 September 2020).

Mari, D. (2019) *Breakfast with the Centenarians: The Art of Ageing Well*. London: Atlantic Press.

Mengers, A. A. (2014) *The Benefits of Being Yourself: An Examination of Authenticity, Unique-ness, and Well-Being*. Online. HTTP: <https://repository.upenn.edu/cgi/viewcontent.cgi?article=1064&context=mapp_capstone> (accessed 5 July 2020).

Moore, T. E. and Mae, R. (2006) Who dies and who cries: Death and bereavement in children's literature. *Journal of Communication*, 37 (4): 52–64.

Newton, E. (1961) Art as communication. *The British Journal of Aesthetics*, 1 (2): 71–85.

Northwestern University (2020) *What Makes Someone a SuperAger?* Online. HTTP: <www.feinberg.northwestern.edu/research/news/podcast/what-makes-someone-a-superager.html#:~:text=Some%20people%27s%20brains%20are%20aging,about%20their%20brains%20and%20lives> (accessed 6 July 2020).

Office for National Statistics (n.d.) *National Life Tables, UK: 2016 to 2018*. Online. HTTP: <www.ons.gov.uk/peoplepopulationandcommunity/birthsdeathsandmarriages/lifeexpectancies/bulletins/nationallifetablesunitedkingdom/2016to2018> (accessed 6 July 2020).

O'Mahony, S. (2016) *The Way We Die Now*. London: Head of Zeus Ltd.

Perry, B., Hogan, L. and Marlin, S. (2000) Curiosity, pleasure and play: A neurodevelop-mental perspective. *Haaeyc Advocate*, 10: 9–12.

Public Health England (2018) *Statistical Commentary: End of Life Care Profiles, February 2018 Update*. Online. HTTP: <www.gov.uk/government/publications/end-of-life-care-profiles-february-2018-update/statistical-commentary-end-of-life-care-profiles-february-2018-update#:~:text=Place%20of%20death,46.9%25%20(Figure%202).> (accessed 14 September 2020).

Ringtved, G. (2016) *Cry, Heart, But Never Break*. New York: Enchanted Lion Books.

Rockwell, J. (1994) *Dennis Potter's Last Interview, on 'Nowness' and His Work*. Online. HTTP: <www.nytimes.com/1994/06/12/arts/dennis-potter-s-last-interview-on-nowness-and-his-work.html> (accessed 8 September 2020).

Shakespeare, W. (2006) *As You Like It*. 3rd Series. London: The Arden Shakespeare.

Stern, Y. (2012) Cognitive reserve in ageing and Alzheimer's disease. *The Lancet Neurology*, 11 (11): 1006–1012. doi.org/10.1016/S1474-4422(12)70191-6.

Stern, Y. (2020) *Cognitive Reserve*. Online. HTTP: <www.ageuk.org.uk/information-advice/health-wellbeing/mind-body/staying-sharp/thinking-skills-change-with-age/cognitive-reserve/> (accessed 11 September 2020).

Sutton-Smith, B. (2008) Play theory: A personal journey and new thoughts. *American Journal of Play*, Summer: 80–123.

The Threshold Choir (2020) *Home*. Online. HTTP: <https://thresholdchoir.org/> (accessed 5 2020).

Twycross, R. (1997) *The Joy of Death*. Online. HTTP: <www.thelancet.com/pdfs/journals/lancet/PIIS0140-6736(97)90053-2.pdf> (accessed 5 July 2020).

Venema, V. (2015) *The People Who Make Last Wishes Come True*. Online. HTTP: <www.bbc.co.uk/news/magazine-34297590> (accessed 13 September 2020).

Wallis, R. (2004) *Why Death Is So Important in YA Fiction*. Online. HTTP: <www.theguardian.com/childrens-books-site/2014/aug/18/death-important-young-adult-fiction-rupert-wallis> (accessed 12 September 2020).

Ware, B. (2019) *Top Five Regrets of the Dying: A Life Transformed by the Dearly Departing*. Carlsbad, CA: Hay House Inc.

Ware, B. (2020) *Regrets of the Dying*. Online. HTTP: <https://bronnieware.com/blog/regrets-of-the-dying/> (accessed 23 September 2020).

Weldon, J. and Weldon, C. (2016) Using play for lifelong learning. In: Tonkin, A. and Whitaker, J. (Eds.), *Play in Healthcare for Adults: Using Play to Promote Health and Wellbeing across the Adult Lifespan*. Oxon: Routledge: 249–262.

Wenk, G. L. (2010) *Why Do Teenagers Feel Immortal?* Online. HTTP: <www.psychologytoday.com/gb/blog/your-brain-food/201008/why-do-teenagers-feel-immortal> (accessed 4 September 2020).

Wheaton, O. (2019) *Where Do Our Sayings for Death and Dying Come From?* Online. HTTP: <www.mariecurie.org.uk/blog/where-do-death-sayings-come-from/259120> (accessed 13 September 2020).

Whitaker, J. and Tonkin, A. (2019) Playful endings. Making meaning at the end of life. In: Tonkin, A. and Whitaker, J. (Eds.), *Play and Playfulness for Public Health and Wellbeing*. Oxon: Routledge.

Williams, A. (2012) *Joy of Death in Bournemouth Aims to Break Taboos*. Online. HTTP: <www.bbc.co.uk/news/uk-england-dorset-19522323> (accessed 6 September 2020).

Yee, H. K., Kin, F. C., Hui, C. W., Jie, T. R. and Peter, D. J. (2019) Dying in cyberworld: Violent video games extinguished children's death concept and attitude. *Southeast Asia Psychology Journal*, 7 (September): 58–69.

York's Dead Good Festival (n.d.) *Home*. Online. HTTP: <www.yorksdeadgoodfestival.co.uk/> (accessed 6 September 2020).

Index

Note: Page numbers in *italics* indicate a figure and page numbers in **bold** indicate a table on the corresponding page.

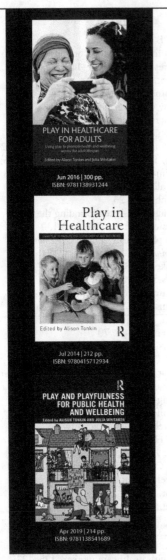

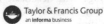

Printed in the United States
by Baker & Taylor Publisher Services